LIVING THERAPY SERIES

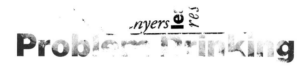

Problem Drinking

A Person-Centred Dialogue

Richard Bryant-Jefferies

D1352345

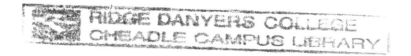
Radcliffe Medical Press

T

Radcliffe Medical Press Ltd
18 Marcham Road
Abingdon
Oxon OX14 1AA
United Kingdom

www.radcliffe-oxford.com
The Radcliffe Medical Press electronic catalogue and online ordering facility.
Direct sales to anywhere in the world.

British Library Cataloguing in Publication Data

A catalogue record for this book is available from the British Library.

ISBN 1 85775 929 X

Typeset by Aarontype Limited, Easton, Bristol
Printed and bound by TJ International Ltd, Padstow, Cornwall

Contents

Foreword

This year marks the centenary of the birth of Carl Rogers, the originator of person-centred therapy and arguably the most influential psychologist of the twentieth century. I have had the privilege of attending many events throughout the world to mark this milestone in the history of the person-centred approach and I have been encouraged and often inspired by the vitality and imaginative innovations of many practitioners. The theory and practice of the approach are evolving in an exciting fashion in the context of a world where all too often the centrality of the client's resourcefulness and of the therapeutic relationship seem to be forgotten in the pursuit of 'quick-fix' solutions and cost-effective procedures.

Richard Bryant-Jefferies' new book is a fine example of the imaginative developments which I have been delighted to witness. It is a truly pioneering venture in a number of ways. In the first place, it demonstrates conclusively the power of the person-centred approach in a notoriously difficult field where, with little justification, directive and behavioural responses have often been deemed the preferred mode of treatment. Secondly, it is, to my knowledge, the first book to offer a meticulously detailed exploration of a complete therapeutic process with a problem drinker. Furthermore, the inclusion of the counsellor's meetings with his supervisor provides a dimension which greatly enriches the reader's understanding of the work and of the immensely demanding challenges involved. Bryant-Jefferies' decision to employ fictitious characters throughout the book not only greatly enhances its value to trainers and trainees, because it permits a focus on key issues, but also lends it the dramatic quality of a novel in the making. Seldom is such profound learning made accessible in so enjoyable a form.

The quality of narrative excitement which permeates the book omens well for the series of which this is the first volume. The intention of Radcliffe's *Living Therapy* series is to enable the reader to enter imaginatively into therapeutic processes and thereby to acquire an experiential knowledge which can seldom be obtained through the more conventional textbook. Bryant-Jefferies succeeds impressively in this aim and, as a result, this book should have a ready readership among not only person-centred trainers and trainees but also among therapists and professionals of other orientations. The subject matter, too, is sadly of such universal significance that the book is likely to win the attention of potential readers outside the United Kingdom.

It occurs to me that the engaging accessibility of the text may also commend this book to those who themselves experience difficulties with alcohol. They may use it either as an adjunct to therapy or as a client self-help manual. I must also confess to some satisfaction at the thought of caring professionals who are not counsellors or psychotherapists being confronted with the advantages and challenges of a regular supervisory relationship. It is to my mind somewhat scandalous that many doctors, social workers and clinical psychologists, for example, are unaccustomed to the consultative support which regular supervision offers and have to make do with perfunctory 'line management' or, in the worst cases, a hurried word with a colleague in the car park or on the way to the canteen. The powerful emphasis on supervision may well prove to be one of the major contributions which the book offers to those many people who attempt to respond to the needs of problem drinkers without benefit of the obligatory supervision relationship which counsellors and psychotherapists enjoy.

The book deserves to be widely read and Richard Bryant-Jefferies is to be congratulated on taking the risk of providing a text which may ruffle a few feathers because it dispels the mystique of the therapeutic enterprise and engages with the person-to-person encounter of counsellor and client and then, for good measure, welcomes the supervisor into the narrative with telling effect. I am certain that Carl Rogers would have smiled on such an intrepid pioneer.

Brian Thorne
Emeritus Professor of Counselling
University of East Anglia
Co-founder, The Norwich Centre
November 2002

Foreword

It is clear that Richard Bryant-Jefferies has extensive experience of work with those who have problems with their use of alcohol: experience gained at all levels of problem drinking from preventative work, with those who still have intact relationships and careers, through to those whose physical and mental health are severely damaged. He describes the realities and pragmatics of dealing with ambivalence and relapse with a clarity that comes from many encounters with those struggling with their use of alcohol.

He consistently conveys a respect for clients both through the collaborative person-centred approach he describes and through his sensitive application of harm-reduction principles. He does not recommend that a client, who has drunk some alcohol, be turned away nor does he see abstinence as the only possible goal. For some, a person-centred\harm-reduction approach is controversial and challenging: the case is convincingly put that this approach is respectful and effective.

In my experience it is rare that a writer combines such an understanding and acceptance of the messiness of alcohol work, a commitment to person-centred counselling and a respect for experimentally derived theories on the course of drinking careers. This integration of sources of knowledge combined with the writer's wide experience makes this a very believable book.

The book is full of useful information for those working with alcohol problems, e.g. on the application of the stages of change model of Prochaska and DiClemente, on when and how to discuss drinking patterns, on how to convey information on alcohol and its effects. I particularly like the approach taken to helping the client appreciate the extent and implications of his drinking.

Above all, the description of the encounters between a counsellor and client and between counsellor and supervisor is drawn from the rich experience of the writer. The method used to convey ideas around these encounters is closer to novels such as *The White Hotel* by DM Thomas than to academic textbooks: for me this is what makes the book come alive and become a compulsive read rather than something to be dipped into as a reference source – it is a gripping story.

This story will be of interest to different groups of readers at many different levels:

- To counsellors – both those in training and experienced, as an account of a series of encounters between a client and counsellor conducted within a person-centred framework.

- To counselling supervisors – the story, on many occasions, identifies and explores processes occurring between counsellor and supervisor, which parallel those between client and counsellor.
- To health and social care workers such as district nurses, practice nurses, GPs, social workers and psychologists. The story is full of information about how to work with the realities of problem drinking, in particular how to clarify drinking patterns and how to prevent and minimise relapse.
- To alcohol workers of all types including those working within the criminal justice system: the interplay between the personal and political issues surrounding our use of alcohol is explored in a low key but insightful way.
- To the general reader – ideas are conveyed in a uniquely stimulating way. This is not a textbook although there is much to learn from it. It is more like an enthralling story with unexpected twists and turns of plot – yet still a believable plot.
- To those experiencing difficulties with alcohol – there are many episodes in this book, which may cause a reader to say 'That is my experience too'.

There are many aspects of this book which are of interest, but two elements seem to me to be of special significance. First, the constant respect which is paid to the client: respect that the client is doing the best they can in the circumstances; respect for the client's choice of drinking goal; and respect for the pace that the client can struggle with difficult issues. Second, the uniquely engaging method used to convey ideas – an intriguing story of an encounter between two people written by someone who has a depth of experience to make the encounter absolutely believable.

Alistair Sutherland
Director, Drug and Alcohol Services
South Staffordshire Healthcare NHS Trust
November 2002

Preface

Few general counselling training courses include a great deal on the subject of working with people with alcohol problems. Yet counsellors and other health and social care professionals are being faced with clients who, for one reason or another, have developed a problematic relationship with alcohol. The counsellor in the GP surgery, the nurse in the accident and emergency department, the social worker concerned with a family, the housing support worker in a city-centre hostel can all expect to encounter people with alcohol problems. I am aware of the growing need for a wider understanding of the issues to be addressed and the ways of working with this client group if we are to ensure that damage is minimised, both to the drinker and to others. Alcohol is, after all, society's favourite drug with its distinctive addictive and mood-altering attributes.

This book sets out to provide material to inform the training process of counsellors and many others who seek to work with this client group. It is intended as much for experienced counsellors as it is for trainees. It provides real insight into what goes on during counselling sessions during a course of therapy for an alcohol-related problem, reflection on the process, and helpful summaries and points for discussion in the wide range of training courses for which it is intended. *Problem Drinking: a person-centred dialogue* will also be of value to the many health-care and social care professionals who are likely to encounter patients or clients, or relatives of these, with alcohol-related problems. For all these professionals, the text demystifies what can occur in therapy, and at the same time provides useful approaches and frameworks that may be used by professionals other than counsellors.

Importantly, I have also written this book for the person who has thought of seeking help for a drinking problem, offering them insight into the process that they might expect in order to resolve their difficulty. There are many myths concerning counselling and I hope that this book helps to reveal to these readers the role of the sensitive and supportive counsellor in this work.

Richard Bryant-Jefferies
November 2002

About the author

Richard Bryant-Jefferies qualified in person-centred counselling in 1994 and remains passionate about the application and effectiveness of this approach. Since early 1995 he has worked at the Acorn Drug and Alcohol Service in Surrey (NHS), introducing a counselling service in GP surgeries for people with alcohol problems. As well as continuing to offer counselling within this specialist arena, he also supervises counsellors who work with people with alcohol problems, works himself as a general counsellor in a GP surgery and offers general counselling supervision.

Richard runs training days on the theme of 'Alcohol Awareness and Response' and has presented his work and ideas at various conferences. He has had articles published in journals (including *BACP*, *HCPJ*, *Practice Nurse*) and had his first book on this topic published in 2001, *Counselling the Person Beyond the Alcohol Problem* (Jessica Kingsley Publishers).

Richard is convinced that the attitudinal values of the person-centred approach and the emphasis it places on the therapeutic relationship are key to helping people resolve not just an alcohol problem, but the issues that generally lie beneath it, fuelling the urge to drink.

Acknowledgements

I would like to thank all the people who offered me support and encouragement when I first started asking what they thought about writing in this way, and those who offered comments on earlier drafts: Moira Plant, Richard Velleman and Brian Thorne. I would also like to thank Deena for allowing me to quote her piece about street drinkers.

I would like to express my sincere gratitude to Maggie Pettifer for her editing skills and her constant enthusiasm for my attempt to bring therapeutic counselling to life for readers.

Introduction

In many ways this book is probably unique, and it is certainly innovative. I have written it to enable the reader to appreciate issues that can arise when working with a person with an alcohol problem, and ways of responding. It is composed almost totally of dialogue between a fictitious client (Dave) and his counsellor (Alan), and between the counsellor and his supervisor (Jan). Within the dialogue are woven the reflective thoughts and feelings of the client, the counsellor and the supervisor.

The dialogue has been written with Alan, the counsellor, applying a person-centred approach (PCA) – a theoretical approach to counselling that has, at its heart, the power of the relational experience to offer growthful influence on the client. The approach is widely used by counsellors working in the UK today: in a membership survey in 2001 by the British Association for Counselling and Psychotherapy, 35.6 per cent of those responding claimed to work to PCA, whilst 25.4 per cent identified themselves as psychodynamic practitioners. The theory underlying PCA is described on page 5.

Many of the responses offered by Alan are reflections of what Dave has said. This is not to be read as conveying a simple repetition of the client's words. Rather, the counsellor seeks to voice empathic responses, often with a sense of 'checking out' that he is hearing accurately what the client is saying. The client says something; the counsellor then conveys that he has heard it, sometimes with the same words, sometimes including a sense of what he feels may be being communicated through the client's tone of voice, facial expression, or simply the atmosphere of the moment. The client is then enabled to confirm that he has been heard accurately, or correct the counsellor in his or her perception. The client may then explore more deeply what they have been saying or move on, in either case with a sense that they have been heard and warmly accepted. To draw this to the reader's attention, I have attempted to highlight the reflection that occurs throughout the work by inserting Alan's reflective thoughts in boxes throughout the dialogue.

The counselling sessions take place within an alcohol counselling agency where the counsellor, Alan, specialises in this area of work. This means that whilst he is there to offer the client the necessary and sufficient conditions for constructive personality change referred to above, and to facilitate the client's process of resolving his alcohol problem, he also has specialist knowledge that at times is offered to the client.

The four supervision sessions are included to offer the reader insight into the nature of therapeutic supervision in the context of the counselling profession, a method of supervising that I term 'collaborative review'. For many trainee counsellors, the use of supervision can be something of a mystery, and it is hoped that this book will go a long way to unravelling this. In the supervision sessions I seek to demonstrate the application of the supervisory relationship. My intention is to show how supervision of the counsellor is very much a part of the process of enabling a client to work through issues and, in this case, come to terms with an alcohol problem.

Many professions do not recognise the need for some form of personal and process supervision, and often what is offered is line management. However, counsellors are required to receive regular supervision in order to explore the dynamics of the relationship with the client, the impact of the work on the counsellor and on the client, to receive support, and to provide an opportunity for an experienced co-professional to monitor the supervisee's work in relation to ethical standards and codes of practice. There are, of course, as many models of supervision as there are models of counselling. In this book the supervisor is seeking to apply the attitudinal values of PCA.

It is the norm for all professionals working in the healthcare and social care environment in the age of regulation to be formally accredited or registered and to work to their own professional organisation's code of ethics or practice. For instance, registered counselling practitioners with the British Association for Counselling and Psychotherapy are required to have regular supervision and continuing professional development to maintain registration. Whilst professionals other than counsellors will gain much from this book in their work with patients or clients with alcohol-related problems, it is essential that they follow the standards, safeguards and ethical codes of their own professional organisation, and are appropriately trained and supervised to work with their clients.

All characters in this book are fictitious and are not intended to bear resemblance to any particular person or persons.

The book is set during the period running up to and after Christmas and New Year, and I have purposefully written it during that period since it is a difficult time for drinkers seeking to change their drinking pattern.

The client, Dave, has contacted the agency as a result of encouragement from his GP. At the start he does not believe that he has an alcohol problem. The first session does not include a lengthy assessment, although many agencies will require this and may include questions concerning drinking history, mental health history and risk assessment, along with questions around the client's social, financial, employment, educational and family background. In my experience, this can get in the way of building the therapeutic relationship and allowing the client to 'tell their story'. Generally I find that much of the information relevant to the client's difficulties is communicated as the session proceeds. In contrast, the often 'question and answer' tone of assessment can set a pattern for the counselling relationship and can have the effect of forcing disclosures from clients before they are ready, or feel trusting of the therapist, to share this information. The power balance in this scenario between counsellor and client is therefore very much biased towards the counsellor. The person-centred approach, on the other hand, seeks to equalise the power balance, for this is a key element of the therapeutic relationship.

This is not a book that sees abstinence as the only response to an alcohol problem. However, I recognise that for many people, abstinence is the only realistic way of ensuring quality of life for the future. I believe in the uniqueness of each individual human being, and that responses must be appropriate to that person's need and experience of using alcohol. For some, an abstinence approach is the best solution; for others, controlled drinking may be more appropriate.

In writing this book, I am mindful that many alcohol problems are not simply about alcohol but are driven by other, deeper psychological needs, often rooted in experiences that have in some way undermined the person's sense of self, or have left them with a strongly adaptive self-concept – the result of negative or inconsistent conditioning in their past.

I hope that I have managed to represent some of the dilemmas, the struggles and the success that can be encountered on the journey towards resolving an alcohol problem. It would be impossible to cover all the angles, but I hope I have included sufficient to communicate the process of counselling a person with an alcohol problem.

Introduction to the person-centred approach

The person-centred approach (PCA) was formulated by Carl Rogers, and references are made to his ideas within the text of the book. However, it will be helpful for readers who are unfamiliar with this way of working to have an appreciation of its theoretical base.

Rogers proposed that certain conditions, when present within a therapeutic relationship, would enable the client to grow towards what he termed 'fuller functionality'. Over a number of years he refined these ideas, which he defined as 'the necessary and sufficient conditions for constructive personality change'. These he described in papers in the late 1950s:

1 Two persons are in psychological contact.
2 The first, whom we shall term the client, is in a state of incongruence, being vulnerable or anxious.
3 The second person, whom we shall term the therapist, is congruent or integrated in the relationship.
4 The therapist experiences unconditional positive regard for the client.
5 The therapist experiences an empathic understanding of the client's internal frame of reference and endeavours to communicate this experience to the client.
6 The communication to the client of the therapist's empathic understanding and unconditional positive regard is to a minimal degree achieved (Rogers, 1957, p.96).

Two years later he further developed his thinking by removing the word 'psychological' from within the first condition. He thereby suggested that what was more important was simply contact, and that this contact may not therefore necessarily need to be psychological. We might therefore conclude that any contact that is qualified by the presence of empathy, unconditional positive regard and congruence has a beneficial and therapeutic effect. At the same time, Rogers dropped 'endeavours to communicate' and rather sought to emphasise how important it is for the client to perceive the 'attitudinal experiences' of the therapist: empathic understanding and unconditional positive regard (Bozarth, 1998).

PCA regards the relationship that we have with our clients, and the attitude that we hold within that relationship, to be key factors. In my experience, many alcohol problems develop out of life experiences that involve problematic relational experiences. These can be centred in childhood or later in life. What is important is that the individual, through relationships that have a negative conditioning effect, is left with a distorted perception of themselves and their potential as a person. I see many people who have learned from childhood experience beliefs such as 'I can never be good enough to be praised for what I have achieved; I never match my parents' expectations', or 'No one was ever there for me when I was hurting; perhaps I am unlovable'. The result is a loss of a positive sense of self, and the individual adapts to maintain the newly learned concept of self. This is then lived out, possibly throughout life, the person seeking to satisfy what they have come to believe about themselves: being unable to achieve, feeling unable to be loved, though perhaps in both cases maintaining a constant desperation to receive what they never had. Yet, perversely, they may then sabotage any possibility of gaining what they want in order to maintain the negatively conditioned sense of self.

How does this kind of experience link to alcohol use? Either the person, perhaps at an early age, discovers that alcohol helps to take the pain away, or perhaps in later life they enter similar experiences of not feeling loved, or not attaining their goals, whereupon the hurt rises to the surface and alcohol is discovered as a means of helping them gain relief. The problem is that respite is temporary and more alcohol is needed to maintain anaesthesia with the risk that prolonged heavy use can lead to dependence and psychological and physical illness.

It is my belief that by offering someone a non-judgemental, warm and accepting, and authentic relationship, the person can grow into a fresh sense of self in which their potential as a person can become more fulfilled. Such an experience fosters an opportunity for the client to redefine themselves as they experience the presence of the therapist's congruence, empathy and unconditional positive regard. This process can take time. Often the personality change that is required to sustain a shift away from alcohol reliance requires a lengthy period of therapeutic work, bearing in mind that the person may be struggling to unravel a sense of self that has been developed, sustained and reinforced for many decades of life.

This is obviously a very brief introduction to the approach. Person-centred theory continues to develop as practitioners and theoreticians consider its application in various fields of therapeutic work. Much has been, and continues to be, written about PCA and a further reading list of suggested titles is included at the end of this book.

Wednesday morning, 11 October

'Hi,' Dave said, rather nervously, as he entered the small and all too cosy room. Two comfortable-looking green chairs, a wooden coffee table with a lamp on it. It wasn't a very bright room, and the chairs looked a bit close.

'Good to meet you,' was the response from a rather too-relaxed looking man in a beige sweater who seemed to be smiling a little too much. 'I'm Alan, glad you made it.'

Dave sat down on the chair by the window, moving it back a little as he did so, and wondered what was going to happen next. He had never been for counselling before, and wasn't really too sure why he was here today. Things had been a little difficult lately and he really wasn't all that sure that he felt comfortable with the idea of coming to counselling. But his doctor had suggested it might be a good idea and, well, he had thought that he might as well give it a go. Now he wasn't so sure. He was aware that it had gone quiet.

'I notice that you are quiet. Ever been to counselling before?' Alan asked.

'No.'

'Can be a bit anxiety-provoking,' Alan commented, sensing Dave's mood and feeling he needed to convey empathy towards what Dave was probably experiencing.

'Yes, feels strange being here. I'm not sure what I am supposed to do.'

'Well, I see counselling as a space for you to explore, to talk about things that may be on your mind, or to express feelings that are present. It is time, your time, to kind of make sense of things perhaps, with someone who has no agenda, no goals other than to allow you to be as you feel you need to be.'

'OK.'

Alan wondered about mentioning how Dave had moved back the chair when he came in, but didn't want to convey any idea that he was analysing his every move. That could have been too threatening. Besides, he was not analysing; he had just noted Dave's movement. It seemed better to just check out if the seating was OK.

'Is it OK for you sitting like this?' he asked.

Dave felt that he was still too close but wasn't at all sure whether or not to say anything. He decided not to. 'Yeah, fine.'

'Sure?'

> Alan really wanted to be sure that Dave felt comfortable, and he knew from his own experience in that training session some years before how the close-ness of the chairs and the angle that they were at could make a profound difference to how people felt. He had certainly been struck by how different he felt when the chairs were too close, or too straight on. He preferred them slightly at an angle, allowing him to feel more free to look away when he felt he needed to. But everyone is different, he thought to himself, and I want Dave to feel at ease with the way he is sitting. He was sensing Dave's discom-fort and wanted to address this.

'I think it is important to be comfortable. How we sit, how close the chairs are can be important. If you want to move your chair please feel free,' Alan suggested.

Dave moved back a little further. 'Thanks. Kind of felt a little crowded.'

'Yes. These are small rooms as well. So, let me say a little about what we offer here and what my role is.'

> Alan then went on to explain about confidentiality, and the limits to that con-fidentiality that were agency policy and professional responsibility. Dave felt OK about this. In fact he was beginning to settle back a little into the chair. Alan explained how the session would last for 50 minutes, and that at the end of this session they could review and discuss what they both felt about working together and, if this was alright, to agree how often to meet up.

'So, how do you want to use our time today? We have about 45 minutes left of the session.'

'I don't know. It's difficult to know where to start. So much has been going on.'

'So many possible starting points, where to begin . . .'

'Yeah. When I phoned a couple of weeks back I had just been to my doctor. I'd been feeling anxious and depressed. Just couldn't seem to get motivated to do anything. She was good, listened to what I had to say, and suggested I get in contact with you. Said she thought my mood could be linked to my drinking. I was a bit surprised that she suggested that.'

'Surprised that she suggested alcohol might be affecting your mood.'

'I don't drink more than my mates do. I don't really understand why she wanted me to come for alcohol counselling.'

'So your drinking seems normal, and you were taken aback by the idea of it being a problem and of coming here?' Alan was aware that he was wondering how motivated Dave was to address his drinking but decided not to comment on this. After all, Dave had not mentioned it himself. It was only a fleeting thought.

Dave felt himself getting a little stronger in his feelings about his drinking not being a problem. 'Yeah, what does she know? I'm drinking the same as everyone else. I don't see why I should be singled out as having a problem.'

Alan noticed Dave's posture tighten; his jaw became a tad more set. 'So you are really not sure that you have a problem. In fact it seems to you that it is not a problem and I sense that it makes you feel a little angry being singled out like this.'

'Yeah, I mean, it really isn't a problem.'

'Your alcohol use is not a problem and it makes you angry when someone suggests that it is.'

'That's right. I get it at home as well. My wife, doesn't like my drinking, says I spend too much time down the pub, or drinking with mates when they come round. I don't see it as a problem.'

Dave was clearly not just talking about feeling angry; he was being it in the room. It is often so important for clients to move from talking about to *being* the feelings that are present for them, and for those feelings to experience warmth and acceptance from the therapist.

'So your drinking is not a problem to you, but it is a problem to your wife.' Alan paused and then added, 'and it makes you angry,' aware that he was leaving it open for Dave to interpret for himself whether he meant the drinking made him angry, or his wife's reaction.

'Bloody angry. I work damn hard all week and a few drinks with my mates are something that I look forward to.'

'Work hard, look forward to a few drinks and . . .'

'Yes, I don't understand why it is a problem.'

'Mhmmm.'

'As soon as I say that I'm off down the pub she starts. "Drinking again, more money pissed up against the wall".'

Alan wanted to just clarify that Dave's wife got angry after the decision to go down the pub. 'So your wife reacts after you have made the decision to go down the pub?'

'Yes, moans about what she has to do in the home, how she never goes out, and God it never ends.'

'She moans at you and you walk out.'

Dave could feel his anger rising, and his frustration. The same pattern time and time again. Why had he married her? Well, he fell for her when she came into his office that day, bringing those papers from the secretarial section. She'd smiled at him, and God she was sexy. He knew he wanted her and he got chatting to her and they started going out. It had been good, bloody good. Then the children were born and somehow things started to change. Dave was not only experiencing his memories, but also feelings associated with them.

Dave suddenly realised he had been so lost in his own thoughts and feelings, he wasn't sure how much time had passed. He looked up. Alan was looking at him.

'You really looked lost in your thoughts then.'

'Yeah, got me thinking.'

Alan felt the atmosphere had changed. Dave didn't seem so angry. Should he mention it? Before he had a chance to decide, Dave continued, 'I was thinking about how it had been with my wife when we first met, you know, how good it was.'

'It was good in the past, at first.'

'Well for some time, really. We met at work. Got on so well, same interests. It just felt so good.'

Alan could sense that Dave was feeling different now. This was a much more reflective Dave sitting before him. Dave's eyes were down, as if he was staring at the carpet, trying to see something that wasn't there. 'You look as if you can still feel those feelings.'

Dave was lost in his memories; images were passing through his mind of 'the good

---

Dave continued to stare downwards in thought. There seemed to be a deep sadness entering the room. It was so, so present. Alan acknowledged it to himself but felt Dave needed to be left in his own world for the moment. He did not want to disturb Dave's flow of feelings. He knew that in therapy it is best to let the client be where they need to be, that the client knows best and that their process can be trusted. The silence continued.

---

times'. He was experiencing feelings he had not felt in years. He had a vague sense that Alan was in front of him, but his focus was on the vividness of what was happening inside him. He heard Alan saying at some point something like, 'I'm here if you want to say something, and I am here if you want to sit with your experiences in silence.' He let the words go by. He was realising how much he wanted the good times back, but they seemed so long ago. He could feel the lump beginning to build in his throat, and before he could do anything to stop it, the tears were welling up in his eyes, hot burning tears that stung and began to trickle down his face. He felt so many feelings, but what stood out was sadness at what he had lost, and fear that it was lost forever.

'Sorry,' Dave said, 'can't help myself.'

'It's OK, seems like you need to let them out.'

Dave took a few deep breaths, wiped his eyes, and a few more deep breaths. He blinked and got a bit of control back. He hadn't expected anything quite like that.

'Where were we?'

'You touched some powerful feelings there. Want to talk about them a little?'

'I was thinking about the good times, and then this feeling of sadness just overwhelmed me, and I felt very frightened.'

'The good times took you into sadness and then it all became very frightening.'

'Yeah,' Dave was looking a little more alert now, 'yeah'. He looked up and caught Alan's eyes. 'I hadn't realised how much I wanted to get our relationship back as it was. That sadness. Like huge waves of it washing over me, through me. I couldn't stand against it.'

'Couldn't stand up to the waves of sadness ...'

'No, they just kept coming, wave after wave. I feel drained. I could do with a drink.'

'That how you usually cope with sadness, go get a drink?'

'I suppose I do, sometimes. Well, makes you feel better, doesn't it?'

Alan sensed Dave's defensiveness but didn't want to push it. He didn't want to confront him. He remembered one of his tutors telling him on his training course: 'If you push the client, they'll push back. You'll end up with a bigger barrier. Give them space. Trust the actualising tendency; it will take them where they need to go. You provide the warmth, the unconditional acceptance that will help them feel safe to challenge their own barriers and defences.'

'Alcohol's a great anaesthetic. Helps you feel better, gets you away from uncomfortable feelings.' Alan responded, sensing that this was going to be an important part of the therapy session.

Dave had come in not seeing his alcohol use as a problem, and it was no good him, Alan, telling Dave it was a problem. Dave had to realise this for himself, to make his own connections and realise what alcohol was doing to himself and to his marriage if it was a significant problematic factor. The truth was that he, Alan, did not yet know the extent of Dave's drinking and what impact it was having. He must not jump to conclusions. Let Dave work it through at his own pace. He will say what he needs to say when the time is right for him to do so. It is not easy for the therapist. Alan could feel the urge to speculate and make connections for Dave, push him. He realised as well the temptation to say something that might make him, the counsellor, appear clever. He mustn't do that (Mearns, 1994). Alan was aware he was losing himself in his own internal battle. He realised it was a supervision issue. He had to put it aside and be there for Dave.

'I suppose so, but sometimes it is just good to have a drink, be sociable, have a few laughs.'

'Mhmmm.'

'Well I think my drinking's not a problem. I enjoy it and I work hard for it.'

Dave has really shifted back into his drinking self, Alan realised, wondering how he had got away from those feelings he was expressing just a short time before. Stay with him. He's doing this for a good reason, probably to avoid those feelings.

'So drinking is not a problem. You enjoy it, and you earn it.'
'That's it.' Dave was looking Alan in the eye and holding the contact.
Alan was aware that he was feeling distinctly uncomfortable. He acknowledged it
   to himself but replied to Dave, 'Not a problem.'
'No.'

Alan was aware that the discomfort was becoming a barrier to hearing Dave. His instinct was to say something. This felt as though it was relevant to the relationship between he and Dave. Experience told him that persistently strong feelings can often be factors that need voicing, making visible, because they often do have significance even if it is unknown at the time.

'Dave, I don't know what this is about, but I have to say that hearing you talk
   in terms of your drinking not being a problem is somehow leaving me feeling distinctly uncomfortable.' He added, 'It may just be me, but I know I am
   wondering . . .'
'Your problem. I'm OK.'
Shit, thought Alan, that hasn't helped. Don't try and debate it. Access Dave's
   view and acknowledge it. Give him space.
'Yeah, OK, maybe it is me. But you're OK with your drinking.'
'Yeah. No problems.'

Stay with him, Alan thought, maybe he's not uncomfortable, or at least not experiencing any tensions that must surely be present if his drinking has been a factor in the changes in his marriage. OK, Alan thought to himself, let's cut out the speculation here. Let's just sit with this. If I speculate too much I'm not in touch with the client, only my own thoughts. I need to be with Dave here. The silence began. Alan felt the presence of a tension, both in the room and he could feel it in himself, a kind of tightness in his lower chest, the kind of sensation that can be around when there are things to be said but which are not being voiced. He waited, aware that Dave was sitting forward again, looking tense. Bodies do give us away, but to say something now about the way Dave's posture seemed so tense, or his own sense of tension, would probably take Dave away from whatever he was dwelling on within himself. Alan simply noted and acknowledged the tension, holding his awareness of its presence.

'Do you think I've got a drink problem?' Dave suddenly asked, looking up and clearly looking as if he wanted an answer and not a reflection.

This is one of those tough moments for the counsellor. Do you reflect the question, or answer it, or try and cover both? The look in Dave's eyes was enough to convince Alan that he knew what to say.

'You really want to know if it is a problem, don't you? My sense is that alcohol use is a problem when it starts causing problems, and these may not always be about quantity, but may be about impact on others' lives. I'm wondering if that's how it is?'

Dave breathed deeply, sucking the air into his lungs, held it and sighed. 'I don't know. It's never felt like a problem to me but ... oh I don't know, there's so much about my life that I don't like, the drinking is the one thing I enjoy and look forward to.'

'The one thing that feels good amongst so many things that you don't like.'

'Yeah, but it shouldn't be like that. I mean, oh I don't know.' There was a short pause, 'It all feels too much.'

'Trying to make sense of it all is just too much.'

'But,' another deep sigh, 'I don't know what to do.' Dave's eyes were watering again; he sat back in the chair looking like a beaten man. He was shaking his head just a little from side to side. 'I don't know what to do.'

Alan sought to let Dave hear what he was saying by reflecting it back. 'I don't know what to do,' saying it in a way that tailed off whilst nodding his head slightly, mirroring Dave's own movement.

Silence settled once more. Dave had so many conflicting feelings and thoughts ripping through him. He knew he had problems in his life, he knew his marriage was going to be on the line if something didn't change, but to admit to having a drink problem? No. He couldn't do that. He wasn't an alcoholic. He only drank what his mates drank. That's not a problem. None of them ever spoke of problems from their drinking. He knew what alcoholics were like, and he wasn't one. He kept saying to himself in his mind, 'I haven't got a drink problem.'

Dave felt a heavy weight in his belly, he felt tense, but he wasn't going to admit to being an alcoholic to himself or to anyone else. He looked at the clock. Ten more minutes. Not much longer to go.

Alan could see Dave's discomfort. Should he say something? He was hesitant in being too empathic to non-verbal impressions in a first session. He remembered how one of his trainers had mentioned some years back how too much empathy too early in the process of building a therapeutic relationship can almost strip a client into a state of psychological nakedness, leaving them feeling highly vulnerable and anxious. Alan wanted to acknowledge his feelings about how Dave was in the moment.

'I want to acknowledge feeling how difficult it can be to face up to such an uncomfortable situation.' Alan hoped this would convey to Dave his sense of the difficulty without making it sound as if he was reading Dave like a book.

Dave heard what Alan was saying. Too right, he thought, what I need is a drink. He said nothing, but continued to stare at the floor, finding himself thinking what a boring colour the carpet was. Grey with flecks in it. Very uninspiring, he thought. Maybe if I just sit here thinking about the carpet those minutes will tick by. Dave had this sense that whatever he said now was likely to lead him into greater discomfort, and he was not prepared to do this. Keep thinking about the carpet, he kept saying to himself. He glanced up at the clock again. Time was nearly up. Need to say something to get out of this. 'Well, I think I've got a lot to go away and think about.'

'A lot to go away and think about?' Alan reflected it as a question and waited, unsure whether Dave might elaborate on exactly what he needed to think about.

'Yeah, I need a bit of time to think about all this.' He looked over at the clock again. 'Time I headed off I reckon.'

Alan was conscious of the time as well, and that Dave had seemed particularly quiet and withdrawn. It hadn't felt like a 'working silence'. He felt Dave had been troubled by what he had experienced during the session and he wanted to respond to that.

'Dave, you may feel a little disorientated given what you have talked about and experienced here this morning and you'll maybe need to look after yourself perhaps when you leave. You have been in touch with some powerful and uncomfortable feelings. You may need to ease yourself back into the world out there. You'll probably be tempted to have a drink. If you do, well, look after yourself.'

Alan knew this was coming from his agenda, but he often offered this view at the end of a first session. He wanted to try and acknowledge what might be happening for his clients, and maybe help them avoid a heavy drinking episode. At the same time, he knew that the clients would do what they needed to do. He felt, however, that what he had said was expressed out of concern and warmth for Dave and his well-being. He wondered whether Dave would want to come back for further sessions.

'You seemed a little distracted during that last silence, but I am wondering if you want to come back and explore this further?' Alan enquired. Dave's internal reaction was swift 'Not bloody likely', he thought to himself, but he said 'OK, how about next week?' A date and a time was agreed and Dave left, pleased to be out in the fresh air as he headed down the road to the Kings Head.

Dave drank heavily the rest of that day. He really wasn't sure why, but he just
needed to. He was feeling so uncomfortable, and when he felt that way he
drank. He got home late that evening and there was a huge row. He ended up
sleeping on the sofa.

Alan was left feeling positive in many ways. He sensed that Dave had
become much more uncomfortable during the session about his drinking
even though he wasn't saying so. Often people do need to feel this discomfort
in order to want to change, but it always brings the risk of increased drinking as well. It is a key part of the application of person-centred theory. The
client is in a state of incongruence, carrying anxiety and tension. Often the
drinking is a way of anaesthetising these feelings but actually it exacerbates
incongruence by distorting experiencing and suppressing the functioning of
the central nervous system (Bryant-Jefferies, 2001). Would Dave return
next week? There was a big risk that he might not. Still, he was open to
being optimistic, knowing that Dave had at one point seriously wanted to
know if he had a problem even though he later moved towards not wanting
to acknowledge this, or maybe he was acknowledging it at some level in
himself but really could not bring himself to voice it.

Summary

Dave has come to the session not believing he has an alcohol problem, and has been allowed to engage with feelings, thoughts and memories that were painful for him to bear. He was allowed to stay with these without being distracted. Alan communicated respect for Dave, giving him time and attention. He sought to reflect his own experiencing where it was felt to be relevant to Dave's process and to empathise with minimal responses to what Dave was saying. Dave is still denying he has an alcohol problem, and he is leaving with an intention not to return but rather to have a drink.

Points for discussion

- Who decides what is the best angle and proximity for the chairs in the counselling room?
- Would it have been helpful for Alan to have asked specifically about Dave's level of drinking?
- What information might Alan have given concerning confidentiality?
- What examples from the text demonstrate the communication of empathy, congruence and unconditional positive regard?
- Can one be over-empathic with a client?
- Does Dave have an alcohol problem?
- What effect might it have had if Alan had said 'yes' to Dave's direct question about whether he has an alcohol problem?
- Should Alan have picked up on Dave's intention not to return, and why might he have *not* sensed this?
- Did Alan really have grounds for his optimism at the end of this session?

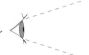

Wider focus

- The arrangement of seating in the room is always important, with consideration for the needs of the client.
- Explaining to the client the nature of, and limits to, confidentiality, which will vary between professions and working settings, is important.
- It is not necessary to push clients, but rather go with them. Avoidance is often for a reason – profound discomfort. Give the client space to explore in their own way and pace, particularly in early sessions.
- Be prepared to question your own reactions to client's material, and seek clarity for yourself, where over- or under-reactions are present, through personal supervision or therapy.

Thursday afternoon, 12 October

The following day Alan was due to go for supervision. This is a requirement for counsellors – an opportunity to reflect on their professional practice and to explore the content and process of their counselling work. Alan's supervisor, Jan, had been a counsellor for over ten years, working in a variety of fields, including substance misuse, and Alan had been going to her for the past three years. In that time they had developed a good, collaborative working relationship.

The idea of supervision as 'collaborative inquiry' (Merry, 1999, p.141) appealed very much to Alan. Alan's view was that the counsellor and supervisor are working in a co-operative relationship to understand what is taking place within both the counsellor–client relationship and the supervisor–supervisee relationship. He felt able to voice his own views, and he was certainly ready to listen to what Jan felt or thought.

Alan had chosen to work with Jan because, like him, she sought to work in a person-centred way. He found it helped him to check out his own practice, and to feel free to speak the same language without having to explain terminology.

Alan had decided he wanted to say a little bit about his session with Dave. He had realised that he had been carrying the intensity of the session with him into the evening that day and it was still very much alive for him as he arrived at Jan's counselling room.

'I saw this new client yesterday and I am still very much with him. I need to describe what happened and try and make sense of it. I'm not sure why it is still with me. It doesn't often happen. I'm sure there's something about this client that is touching into my own stuff.'

Jan knew Alan well enough to trust his judgement about his own needs. She invited him to say more.

Alan described the session. He highlighted the silences, the distress that Dave had shown towards his marriage, and his wanting to know if he had a drink problem – a question that somehow never really got answered although he, Alan, suspected that a process was running inside Dave which was going to lead him towards making his own realisation about this. Alan could feel a blank inside himself and said 'I don't know'. He then smiled to himself, thought for a moment, and said, 'That's interesting. Dave said, "I don't know" a few times. I think I'm parallel processing here. I think his sense of "I don't know" is with me as well.'

It is not unusual for process in the counselling session to be carried into supervision. The sense of 'I don't know' was very much present in the super-vision. Jan could also feel a sense of not knowing what to do with this client, and voiced this. They agreed that it somehow felt important to have made this visible in supervision. One of the aspects of supervision that Jan and Alan both agreed on was that work done in supervision also impacted in some way on the client even before the client was next seen. This may seem strange, but they had both experienced situations with clients where subject matter discussed in supervision and insight gained as a result seemed to coincide with similar insights being gained by the client. They realised not everyone saw it this way, but they both felt that some kind of connection with the client existed whilst they discussed what had been happening in the counselling session.

'I am aware as well of wondering where Dave is on the "cycle of change" model,' Alan commented.

This is a model devised originally in the early 1980s by two American psy-chologists (Prochaska and DiClemente, 1982) to describe the process and stages people pass through when undergoing change. It has been updated recently, although many people still refer to the original form. Basically, the model suggests that people pass through stages. Each stage has certain characteristics and demands particular areas of focus and response in order to help the client move on.

There is the stage of *pre-contemplation* in which the client is not thinking about change; *contemplation*, where the client is in the process of think-ing about change, exploring it, weighing it up; next, at least in a more recent version, there is a period of *preparation*, where change is prepared for and planned; then there is an *action* phase, where the planning is acted on; then comes a period of *maintenance*, with the planned change being maintained; finally there is a stage of *lapse or relapse* which may or may not happen, although often it does and is part of the learning curve.

Clients may exit the process as well, either in contemplation or prepara-tion, if they feel that the time is not right for change, or simply find them-selves unable to sustain their motivation. They may exit from maintenance, having achieved their goal – whether that is reduction or abstinence – and move on from being so 'alcohol-centred' in their lives. Finally, they may exit from lapse or relapse, going back into their previous pattern of drinking.

Alan reflected for a moment or two and a thought crossed his mind that he hadn't really considered before in relation to this model. 'You know, it's as if there are parts of Dave that are in pre-contemplation and other parts that are definitely in contemplation.'

Jan was intrigued, 'Can you say a little more about this?'

'Well ... Dave, when he was saying "Do you think I have a drink problem?" sounded as though he really felt he did have a problem, and wanted to do something about it. He never actually said this, but on reflection after the session, and sitting here now, I have a real sense that part of him knew he had a problem.'

'Can we define that part in some way?'

'I'm not sure, but it seemed to be linked to a sad part of himself that was so upset when he was thinking back to how his marriage had been in the early days. I think that aspect of his nature really wanted to change, but it was also so uncomfortable for him to be with that part of himself.'

'I can feel a sense of loneliness in that struggle to be with that sadness.'

'That was a word that was never used, but I think you are right, there was a profound sense of loneliness, and maybe that will be explored another time. I wasn't picking it up at the time, but now it makes a lot of sense. Why wasn't I picking it up?'

'You wonder why you weren't picking it up in the session and I am left wondering what loneliness means for you in your experience?'

'Oh-oh. That's the link. Since being on my own after my relationship break-up last year I have certainly had some feelings of loneliness. I guess being at home yesterday evening, I didn't have anything planned, I was having a quiet night in, I guess it stuck with me more.'

'So maybe Dave's unvoiced loneliness touched your own sense of loneliness and those feelings became more present for you.'

'Yeah, that really does make sense. I thought I had moved on from those feelings. It's amazing how you carry them with you. It's a damned good job I come to supervision. You picked it up.'

'I think sometimes elements of the therapy don't get seen by the therapist. They can be too involved to register everything. I see myself as being here to catch whatever has passed through you without impression and hopefully draw attention to it. It's a mixture of empathy and congruence on my part: empathy towards what you are describing in terms of the session and how you experienced it and are experiencing it as you tell me, and congruence as I seek to note my own reactions and to communicate what becomes present for me.'

'You really do use yourself in supervision, which of course we do in therapy as well, particularly because we work with the person-centred approach.'

'In the final analysis, the one resource we have is ourselves. It is us that we bring into therapeutic relationships with our clients. The more present we can be, the more complete the relationships we can establish, the greater the likelihood that the client will engage more fully with their own selves and move from incongruence towards greater congruence. You know that though.'

'Yes, but it is important to be reminded of it!'

'So how are you feeling towards Dave now? It feels to me as though something has shifted, it feels less heavy in some way.'

'Yes, it does seem as though we have allowed more of Dave to become present here. I have this crazy image of him sitting somewhere and suddenly feeling a little more aware of himself.'

'It's a nice thought, but it could be fantasy too.'

'We may never know, but I feel much more freed up to work with Dave now. In fact I am aware of a powerful contrast to when I came in here this afternoon. I'm sure I wasn't looking forward to working with Dave, but now I feel more drawn to wanting to help him. I'm sure it's that loneliness issue. I didn't want to get too close to him because at some level I knew it would demand of me to get close to an aspect of myself that is uncomfortable. I'm going to explore this further in my own therapy. I don't know that it is appropriate to keep focusing on it here, I have some other clients I want to talk about this afternoon.'

'Will you be having a therapy session between now and when you are next due to see Dave?'

'Yes, Monday evening. I see Dave again late Wednesday morning.'

> The supervision continued with a focus on some of Alan's other clients. As he left, Alan was aware of the shift. He could think of Dave but it was lighter, he could reflect on him without feeling stuck with him. It seemed that no matter how much therapy and personal development work you did, there were always aspects of oneself that clients could hook into, and he was so grateful both for his sake, and for Dave's, that he attended supervision of a kind that explored not only the content but also the process of counselling. He had had 'clinical' supervision and 'management' supervision in the past, but neither really satisfied his need to reflect on the process of being in therapeutic relationships with clients. He also valued Jan's openness to accepting and offering not only cognitive perspectives but also much more subjective, intuitive and emotional responses as well, one of the principles of 'collaborative inquiry' (Merry, 1999).

Summary

Alan has clarified and deepened his sense of Dave. He has been given time and space to explore the session and his reactions and interventions. He has linked his experience to theoretical ideas related to the cycle of change. Alan has also recognised an issue for personal therapy with regard to 'loneliness'.

Points for discussion

- How has the supervision session informed Alan's practice?
- How do you think you would feel having Jan as your supervisor?
- Does the word 'loneliness' that Jan voiced seem to you to have application to Dave?
- How important is personal therapy for counsellors and other professionals who seek to work with therapeutic issues?
- How would supervision of this kind be of value in settings other than counselling?

Wednesday morning,
18 October

Alan looked at the clock, it was 11.00 am and Dave was due any moment for his session. He sat quietly, seeking to hold himself open. He did not want to hold any preconceived ideas; he wanted to be fresh to connect with Dave when he arrived and to continue the process of building a therapeutic relationship. He noted that he really wanted Dave to arrive. He had really felt moved by how Dave had been in that first session, the struggle that had seemed to be taking place inside him. Would he return? The intercom sounded. Dave had arrived. 'I think he's had a drink,' was the comment made by the receptionist.

Alan wasn't surprised. It must have been difficult for Dave to come back, and probably he felt he had needed a drink to calm some of his anxieties. Well, we'll soon find out. Alan went out to find him.

'Hi Dave, come on through.'

'Thanks.' Dave avoided eye contact. It had been a struggle to come. He really had some mixed feelings about all this. He had felt very uncomfortable at the thought and decided on the way to just drop into the off-licence and get a can of lager, nothing too strong, 5% stuff, but enough to take the edge off it all. Anyway, he was here now and wondering what he was going to talk about. It had been a hell of a week.

'So, glad you made it back, not always easy.'

'Nearly didn't make it. Wasn't sure about coming. Felt so bad after last time. Wasn't sure I could face that again.' Dave wondered if Alan had noticed he'd had a drink.

'So you had a bad time after the last session?'

'Yeah, went straight down the pub for a couple of beers. Didn't go into work in the afternoon, phoned them to say I wasn't well. They seemed OK about it.'

'Mhmmm.'

'Not sure what to say. Had a blazing row when I did get home. It's not been easy all week. My wife, Linda, hasn't really let up, and so I've been down the pub every night. Been a bit drunk a few times, I can tell you.'

'Blazing row, down the pub every night, drunk a few times.'

'Yeah, difficult week.' Dave sat silently and waited for Alan to respond.

> As Alan finished his reflection he had suddenly been struck with the aware-
> ness that he had no idea exactly how much Dave drank. Maybe this was
> the time to introduce it? He didn't like to push it too quickly. Sometimes it
> was better to begin building the relationship before exploring what was
> being drunk.
>
> He heard Dave say it had been a difficult week but he was stuck with this
> wonder about how much Dave was drinking. It felt very present and he was
> aware of the silence. He decided to voice it and to own it. He had learned not
> to ask how much. Few heavy drinkers can accurately recall exactly how
> much they have been drinking, but they know what brand or type of alcohol
> they generally drink. Best to go in on what kind of drink and then gradually
> build up the picture.

'Dave, I've really heard you say that it has been a difficult week, and you may
   want to keep a focus on that. But I am very conscious of sitting here wondering
   what it is you usually drink.'

'Usually lager in the pub, nothing too strong, it's what we all drink.'

'So on an average evening you'd be drinking pints pretty constantly till closing
   time, in rounds presumably?'

'Yeah.'

'So how many would you generally get through of an evening?'

'Depends really, but I reckon about six to eight pints.'

> Alan started doing the mental arithmetic. Half a pint of lager was equal to
> one unit, so six to eight pints meant 12 to 16 units during the evening. This
> was a lot, certainly above safe drinking for a man, which is three to four
> units a day. He decided not to mention this yet. He didn't want Dave to
> become defensive. He wanted to try and get the whole drinking picture
> first. Alan did not ask directly *how much* Dave drinks, but has sought to
> encourage him to give a general picture of his drinking pattern with a
> focus more on *what* he drinks and *when*. He has found this to be generally
> more accurate.
>
> The assessment of alcohol use has been emphasised by Velleman (2001),
> along with methods for obtaining this information. He also draws attention
> to the fact that the interaction between counsellor and client should not be
> inquisitorial, quoting Rollnick *et al.* (1999, p.113): 'It is a conversation, not
> an investigation'.

'Ever drink anything else in the pub?'

'Might have a Scotch to end the evening.'

'Double?'

'Usually. Well, singles are hardly worth bothering with, are they?'

'Single doesn't really have much effect for you?'

'No.'

Another two units, as a single measure of spirits equals one unit. 'And this is every night?'

'Pretty much. Sometimes I might stay in, but then I'll usually make sure I've got some cans, half a dozen usually.'

'What, the middle-of-the-road lagers, 5% or so?'

'Yeah, I think it's about that. Not the really strong stuff, that 9% stuff is awful. You've got a real problem if you drink that. But I don't, so it's not a problem.'

'So as long as you keep off the strong lager it really doesn't seem much of a problem?'

'Yeah. Keep to normal lager, that's me, can't go wrong with that.'

Alan made a note of Dave's attitude towards the strong lagers. He might need to mention that later when they got into looking at the total amount Dave was drinking.

'Any spirits at the end of the evening when you drink at home?'

'Yeah, usually have a couple of Scotches. Sets me up for sleeping.'

'Larger ones than you have in the pub?'

'Maybe.' Dave was beginning to feel suspicious. This felt like he was being interrogated a bit. Alan sensed the change in Dave and decided to comment. 'You're looking a bit troubled. I really only need to try and get an idea of what you're drinking so we can begin to make sense of your drinking pattern. We rarely stop and think about how much we drink, particularly when we drink with other people, or when we have been drinking a particular way for some time.'

'Well, I was wondering where we were heading with all the questions.'

'Yeah, OK. Bit of a sensitive topic given that you've had a bit of a heavy week. Where do you think the questions were leading?'

'I don't know. Just felt a bit uncomfortable, you know?'

'What, talking about how much you drink leaves you feeling uncomfortable?'

'Yeah.'

'Mhmmm.'

Alan decided to let this moment hang in the air, let Dave just feel that discomfort a bit more before commenting. He knew that people tend to change things because they feel uncomfortable. Change happens either because someone wants to get away from discomfort, or they have experienced something more pleasant that they want more of. He was concerned about Dave's drinking. He was clearly drinking close to 20 units a day, and if he had been maintaining this for some time, then he was likely to be dependent. And he hadn't explored what else Dave might be drinking. He'd had one this morning – well, he could smell alcohol as Dave had come into the room. Was that a routine drink, a morning habit, or just because of coming here?

'I'm aware that it smells of alcohol in here, wondering whether this is the effect of your drinking last night or if you had a quick one this morning on the way in.'

'Nothing since last night.' Dave realised he was feeling ashamed at having had the can that morning. He didn't want to admit to it. He didn't want Alan to know.

'OK. Just aware of an alcoholly smell in the air. Sometimes it can come in on peoples' clothes. People don't realise that if they drink heavily, even if they try to get the smell off their breath, their sweat carries an alcohol odour.'

He was sure Dave had had a drink but he was going to accept that Dave needed to say no for his own reasons. Some would argue it needed challenging, but as a person-centred counsellor he was willing to accept what Dave needed to say. If Dave was right, then fine. If he wasn't being honest, well Dave knew that, and maybe he didn't trust him enough to say it, or maybe he was feeling too uncomfortable. Alan let it go. It didn't matter. Dave didn't seem alcohol-affected in how he was behaving, and he certainly was happy to see him even though he may have had a drink. To only see people who were dry on the day meant that those who needed a drink to come might never get a service. He recognised how important it was that he had worked through his thoughts on this and was clear on his boundaries (Bryant-Jefferies, 2001).

'So, just to help me get a clear picture, let's recap. Six to eight pints of lager most evenings plus a double Scotch when you are in the pub in the evening. Six cans of lager plus a couple of large Scotches when you stay in.'

'That's right.'

'You don't drink regularly at any other times, just in the evenings?'

'No, well I may have the odd pint at lunch times, but that's not a real drink, just something to have during the lunch-break.'

'Not a real drink, I hear what you say, but it is still alcohol going through the body. Is this every day?'

'Pretty much.'

Alan was getting concerned. This sounded like dependence. He really needed to check this out a little more. Dependence, he knew, was likely at this level of intake, the body needing a top-up because otherwise it would begin to withdraw which, with alcohol, can be life-threatening. In extreme cases people would fit, have seizures, hallucinate. It really was a serious issue.

'Dave, this may seem an odd question, but I'm curious as to how you feel before that first drink at the end of the morning. Ever feel on edge, a bit short tempered, finding it hard to feel settled or to relax?'

'Funny that, yeah, I do. By about 11 o'clock I'm usually keeping an eye on the clock. We head off around 12.00. The pub's round the corner.'

'Couple of pints?'

'Yeah, two or three.'

Right, Alan thought, I need to say something to him about how much he is getting through. It is a damaging level and it does sound as though he is showing signs of dependence. He doesn't appreciate the damage that might occur and out of respect for him I want to help him appreciate this. One last question though. 'Ever have a day when you don't drink?'

'No, can't remember when I had a day without a drink.'

'OK, so let's look at this in terms of units. Have you come across the idea of units of alcohol and safe drinking?'

'No.'

'Well, not everyone is aware of it, but there are recommended limits to drinking insofar as it affects people's health. And the way alcohol intake is measured is by units. One pint of ordinary strength lager is about two units; a single measure of spirits is one unit. Yeah?'

'OK.'

'So I estimate you are drinking around 18 to 24 units a day; 14 to 18 units in the evening and four to six units at lunch times.'

'Is that a lot?'

Recommended safe drinking is three to four units a day, which is a couple of pints of lager, maximum.'

'What! Come on.' Dave looked disbelieving. 'That's nothing, I mean, we are drinking that in the first hour of a session, sometimes the first half hour.'

'Yeah, it doesn't sound much, but that is what is recommended. I really am concerned, Dave, you may not feel it, but you are drinking enough to be doing damage to your health.'

'But I never feel really drunk. I'm never ill with it.'

'Not feeling drunk isn't a good sign. I'm not just saying that, it's true. You get tolerant to alcohol. You don't feel the effect the same.'

'But it doesn't feel like a problem. It's what I do, have been doing for years. I can't just stop. I don't want to stop.'

'Yeah, it doesn't feel like a problem and no one's asking you to stop. What I am saying is that you are drinking at a level that is damaging and you are probably experiencing signs of dependence, of needing a drink to stave of feeling a bit shaky, on edge. Ever sweat heavily in the night?'

'Yeah, every night.'

'And you've been drinking at this level for years now?'

'Last few years, I suppose since I was 25. Previously I didn't drink at lunch times, and maybe had three to four pints in the evenings. Well, I was doing other things then, I had only recently met my wife.'

Dave was getting worried. Alan seemed to him to be pretty assured about what he was saying. 'You do think I've got a drink problem, don't you?'

No point in reflecting this one, thought Alan, got to be honest, I owe it to him. I want to be honest, and I have to be congruent if I am to help him become more congruent in this relationship. He looks serious and I sense he wants a straight answer.

'Yes.'
The word hung heavily in the air and the silence that followed was intense.
'What do I do?'
'What do you want to do?'
'You really think it's a problem. You really think I ought to cut back?'
'I do, but I want you to think about it because it is a big part of your life.' Alan knew that people who rushed into changing a drinking pattern without thinking it through often found themselves unable to sustain the change. He wanted Dave to give it thought and explore the situation he found himself in.
Dave was stunned. He didn't want to believe any of it, but somehow there was something about Alan that he trusted. He wasn't telling him what to do, but he seemed to be being up front about things. But he had never thought of his drinking as a problem. His mates all drank. He went to work each day. He didn't feel ill. He never had hangovers.
'Are you sure about all this, I mean, really sure?'
'I'm afraid so, Dave. You are drinking heavily and I think you need to be aware of this and to think about it.'
'But I'm not an alcoholic.'
'Sounds a pretty strong affirmation, "I am not an alcoholic".'
'Well, I'm not, am I? How do you see my drinking then?'
'I think of you as a heavy drinker certainly, and that given the amount you drink you are at serious risk. I was going to say at serious risk of developing a drink problem, but in many respects alcohol use is already causing some problems, for instance, at home, and drinking at the level that you are doing is putting your health at risk. And I want to acknowledge that not everyone finds the label "alcoholic" an easy one to bear. It's a label that troubles you, isn't it?'

Alan could sense Dave's unease about this word 'alcoholic'. It was so loaded, and so associated in many people's minds with really extreme drinking. Some people found the label helped, gave them a sense of identity. If they got to AA they could find their kindred spirits and a sense of being part of a caring and supportive family that many members had never really had. Others did not want the label and felt much more able to accept that they were 'a person with a drinking problem'. Often problem drinking is a learned behaviour or a kind of coping strategy to deal with emotional hurt.

'It does trouble me. I don't want to be an alcoholic. I see them down by the river every day. I'm not like them.'

'That sounds pretty clear: you don't want to be like them, you don't want to be an alcoholic.'

'But you think I am.'

'I think you've got a drink problem, and if you carry on as you are you are at risk of being with them.'

'But I've got a job, my marriage, my house, my children.'

'Yes, you have got all these things, and I can sense how important they all are for you.' Alan really felt for Dave as he tried to make sense of it all, and he knew he just had to add something to that last sentence. He really wanted Dave to be aware of what was at risk, 'And many of the people you see by the river had them once as well'.

'Serious?'

'Yeah, I know some of them, I have heard their stories.'

Alan had worked with some of the street drinkers and had listened to some horrendous stories. He didn't see them as people to look down on or avoid. He had touched and been touched by their human qualities. So many of the street drinkers he knew were incredibly sensitive – well, actually he found sensitivity to be a characteristic of most people who had drinking problems. Whether it was genetic or environmental, so many of the drinkers he knew were extremely sensitive emotionally, easily moved to tears, easily hurt, and they had found alcohol brought them temporary relief. Of course, it was only temporary. One of his clients had written down some thoughts. He could remember how her words had touched him deeply.[1] She was 41 and had been in two children's homes, two boarding schools and with two sets of foster parents, and had got into drinking for various reasons, but particularly home problems. So many people developed alcohol problems as a result of using alcohol to try and solve problems. Heavy alcohol use is never a safe long-term solution to anything.

The other characteristic he had seen time and time again among heavy drinkers was the presence of loss in their lives, often really significant

---

[1] 'I know most of those who do drink on the streets. I feel sorry for them because they do not ask to be in that situation and I have sat with them [in local towns] for a drink and I have heard people say things like, "they are a waste of space" and "need locking up and throw away the key". They are human just like me and other people. All they want is to be wanted and loved and liked. So instead of saying things like that, let them know that people care. I love them all and they care for me, and if you talk to them they make you feel safe. It is alright for other people to say that there is a light at the end of the tunnel, but if you are sleeping on the streets, that is all of us drinkers, see. So next time when you are shopping for food and other things just stop and think about them. We are good people.'

losses. Whether this had contributed to their sensitivity, or just happened to be how it was, varied from person to person. But it was usually there. Losses in childhood were many: those resulting from the death of a close relative; loss of childhood and innocence due to abuse – physical or sexual; loss of friends, perhaps, where there were lots of moves of house; loss of any feeling of security where parents were unpredictable, maybe drinking themselves. It went on into adulthood as well: loss of a marriage, of access to children, of a job, a house, friends. So much problem drinking seemed connected to losses of one kind or another. Alcohol, nature's anaesthetic, but did it have a sting in the tail if you took too much!

'I've got to do something, cut back somehow. I can't see myself stopping,' Dave continued, feeling a little resentful at the idea of having to never have another drink, and somewhat shocked that Alan was saying that he might lose everything.

'Don't stop, you might withdraw. In fact it is highly likely you would withdraw. Best to try and cut back slowly. If it gets too much then we talk to your GP and see what medication can be prescribed to help you.' Alan was aware of just how dangerous it could be to just stop, particularly when the drinker is dependent. It could be life-threatening.

'I need to do something. How about if I try to knock out the odd pint?'

'Yeah. Any particular one?'

'Maybe go down the pub a little later?'

'Going down the pub later may well work.'

Alan was aware that Dave was moving not only into contemplating change but wanting to take action. He really had been affected by the discussion they had been having. But he wanted Dave to plan it, take his time, not rush into anything too dramatic and get a bad reaction. He realised he had been a bit hard, bringing in a little bit of an extreme view, although in all honesty he knew it wasn't extreme, it was a genuine risk, and it was a view that he was experiencing in response to what Dave had said. He wasn't offering this view simply as a technique to motivate Dave to change. This was one way in which the person-centred approach could be seen to differ from 'motivational interviewing', used widely in addiction counselling (Miller and Rollnick, 1991). The motivational interviewer will intervene specifically to motivate change. The person-centred counsellor does not have this agenda, but responds congruently and out of respect for the client's well-being. The fact is that people do lose everything through alcohol, and coming from all walks of life.

'What else can I do?'

'What do you think would help?' Alan wanted Dave to try to plan changes for himself rather than offer him ideas that might be unrealistic for him and not the result of his own inner urge to change his drinking pattern.

'I feel I need to take it slowly. Just take it one step at a time and see how it goes.' Dave was aware of feeling a mixture of wanting to show he had control over his drinking by cutting back dramatically, and of feeling a distinct uneasiness at the idea and whether he could actually manage it. He said nothing, but was aware of not feeling at all comfortable.

'Take it slowly, one step at a time.' Alan was aware that he was wondering about Dave completing a drinking diary. It was an old and well-tested method of helping someone to raise awareness of their drinking pattern.

'One idea that has been around for a while, and which can prove helpful, is to keep a diary of what you're drinking as you go through the week, and look for opportunities to cut back a little each day as you get a feel for your pattern and when you might be able to knock out the odd drink. I've got some sheets that you can fill in. There are columns for when you start drinking, who with, how you're feeling before and after, how much you drink. Help us both get a really clear picture of what's going on. It will help you to make sense of it a little more and give us a basis to work from. It's an idea that's been around for a while. I'm not saying do it; I'm saying it's something many people have found useful.'

'Yeah, that makes sense. Look I need to go and think about all this. I need some time to reflect on it all, time to be on my own.' Dave lapsed into silence. He was aware that he had said he needed to time to think last week, but somehow he felt different this time. He wasn't sure why. He felt somehow more aware that he did have to think seriously about his drinking. Alan seemed pretty genuine. He didn't seem to pull any punches, but he also seemed genuinely concerned.

'Time on your own . . . ,' Alan responded.

Dave remained silent for a short while again. He was thinking about why he was feeling different, why he was taking Alan seriously. He realised what it was, not being judged. I don't feel he's judging me. But it is leaving me judging myself. He took a deep breath and his thoughts went to home and to his mates. What was he going to tell them? He looked up. 'What do I tell people? How will my mates react? What do I tell my wife, she's married to an alcoholic?'

Alan was aware of the look of concern that had swept across Dave's face. 'What to tell people or how much to tell people, and who do you tell. And particularly what do you tell your wife. What do you want her to hear, Dave?'

'I have to tell her I have a problem but that I am trying to deal with it. I have to tell her I'm trying to cut back. No, I'm going to cut back.' Dave looked at the clock.

Alan noticed his glance.

'What do you tell them? What do you want to tell them?'

'That's what I have to think about. I do need to talk to Linda.'

Alan glanced up at the clock. It was nearly time to draw to an end. 'I'm aware that you have a difficult decision to make about who to tell and what to say, and I am aware that our time is nearly up today.'

'Yeah, I need to think this through for myself. You mentioned something about diaries earlier?'

'Yes, take these diaries, take some time to think and when you come back next week we'll maybe explore your options, or whatever you feel you need to talk about when you arrive. It's your time, bring whatever you want here.'

Dave nodded. 'Yeah. I need to speak to my wife. I don't suppose she could come along next time to hear what we have been talking about. I mean I think she'd understand more listening to you. I don't think she'll listen to me.'

'Scary to tell your wife these things, not knowing how she will react. How about you have a chat with her, and if you both agree, then come along together next time. If you can give me a ring and let me know, that would be helpful. I leave it up to you.'

'OK. Same time, same day next week?'

'Yes, 11.00 am next Wednesday. See you then. Take care of yourself.'

'Yeah. I feel a lot different to how I did at the end last week. I just had to have a drink then. I feel very different today, very different.'

'Different?'

'Yeah, much more thoughtful. I have a lot to think about. I have to make some changes to my drinking and I'll keep a record. See you next week.'

Alan sat back in the chair after Dave had gone and reflected on the session. It had been intense and although there wasn't much talk or exploration of feelings, they were certainly very present in the room. It had felt right to focus in on exactly what Dave was drinking. It had been a shock for him, but that shock was bound to happen if he was going to address his alcohol use. Alan could only hope that it was timely. He decided to go out for a five-minute walk to get some fresh air and to clear his head. He remembered that he had never said anything about Dave having come in having had a drink. Then he remembered, of course, Dave had denied it. Probably felt ashamed. No one likes admitting to something they're ashamed of, he thought. Why should we treat people with alcohol problems any different, calling it denial and making it seem bad. It was part of being human.

He'd never had a problem either seeing people who had had a drink before the session. So long as they are not completely out of it or their behaviour threatening, Alan would happily see clients who were alcohol-affected. He had heard people say this was colluding, but for Alan people chose to drink, like any other choice, for a reason. He didn't want to turn them away. It was important for him to acknowledge the person beyond the alcohol problem, and so long as it seemed there was psychological contact and he did not feel threatened or unsafe, he would see people who had been drinking. And, of course, for the dependent drinker it was impossible for them to get to him without having alcohol in their bodies. A no-alcohol policy would have simply discriminated against the most needy group of drinkers.

Dave went and sat in the park, he needed time to think. He wasn't sure what he would do next, but he knew he needed to make some changes. He lost track of time as he pondered on what had just occurred in the session. He had a problem. He'd known it before but wasn't prepared to face it. Now it felt as if he had no choice. He didn't want to lose everything, but he knew as well that it was possible. Things had been difficult at home recently, and his wife had threatened to throw him out on more than one occasion, or leave herself. Oh well, he thought, time to head back to work. I think I need to be a little more aware of what I'm doing and start making a few more healthy choices in my life. The sun was shining, it felt warm on his face as he walked along the path back to the High Street and the office where he worked. Things have to change, he thought, they *have* to. He suddenly realised he felt very alone facing this problem. It seemed huge. He could feel himself becoming incredibly anxious inside, and he felt himself sweating although he was aware of feeling cold. He was just passing the pub . . .

Summary

Dave finds it difficult coming to the session, but he makes it although he has needed a can of lager to get himself there, which he denies having had when Alan raises the issue. The pattern of Dave's drinking is raised by Alan, who later introduces 'units of alcohol'. It becomes clear Dave is probably drinking dependently. He is advised not to just stop. Dave realises that he is beginning to respect Alan and it is linked to Alan's honesty. He raises the issue of bringing his wife to a session. The idea of Dave completing a drinking diary is introduced.

Points for discussion

- How can Alan justify raising the question of what and how much Dave drank in the way, and at the time, that he did?
- How do you feel about safe drinking and raising the issue with a client?
- Should clients who are to some degree alcohol-affected be given counselling?
- Should a counsellor challenge a client when they believe their client has been drinking?
- Alan tells Dave that he thinks he has an alcohol problem. Was this appropriate and justified as a congruent response?
- What do you feel about street drinkers? How would you react if a street drinker were referred to you as a client?
- Should Alan see Dave and his wife together and what would be the pros and cons of agreeing to this?
- What should be included in a drinking diary? And why?

Wider focus

- The matter of whether or not to work with clients who have had a drink, or are clearly alcohol-affected, is one that affects all helping professions, and it is important for all professionals to have thought through their response and understand their reasoning.
- Whether a drinking behaviour is problematic or not is an issue for everyone. Clients may listen to someone who they respect, but sometimes it is more helpful to encourage the client to think about the effects of their drinking and ask themselves the simple question, 'does my drinking cause or threaten to cause me or others problems?'
- It is dangerous for a dependent drinker to just stop. They should never be advised to do this, and if they plan to then they should consult their GP or a specialist alcohol service first.

Wednesday morning, 25 October

Dave did not arrive. Alan was feeling concerned. Whilst he appreciated that Dave had every right to make his own choices, he was worried about what might have happened over the previous week. Dave had reached a point of realising he had a problem, or at least he was certainly moving that way, but how was he going to react to this on his own, or back with his mates, or at home? Alan hadn't had a phone call so he didn't know whether or not Dave had talked to his wife about them both coming.

Time passed. Alan reflected on that last session. Could he have said something more? Did he miss something? As usual the tempting thoughts were around what he might have 'done'. He smiled as he realised where his thoughts had taken him. What was it Carl Rogers had written? Oh yes: 'Therapy is not a matter of doing something to an individual, or of inducing him to do something about himself. It is instead a matter of freeing him for normal growth and development' (Rogers, 1942, p.29).

Somewhere out there Dave was making choices, the best he could make for himself given his situation. Maybe his situation had changed, maybe he had had further problems related to his drinking? Alan did not have answers. Time passed. Twenty minutes had now gone by and still no sign of Dave. OK, he thought, I'd better get a letter to him, let him know I'm concerned and offer him another appointment for next week.

Dave had had a bad week. After sitting in the park thinking, he just began to feel overwhelmed by a sense of loneliness as he walked back to work. He felt so ashamed and didn't really want to tell anyone about the fact that his drinking was a problem. He knew he ought to tell his wife, but how would she react? How would he feel? Just now he knew he felt awful. He went for a drink, and another, and ended up in the pub all afternoon and into the evening. It helped him stop feeling.

He arrived home late. The door was locked. He tried getting in, started shouting, broke a window in his frustration. The police were called and he was arrested and spent a night in the cells. It was a long, lonely night. He got some sleep but on awaking he hadn't a clue where he was or why he was there. The police explained to him what had happened. He could remember nothing. He couldn't believe it, but he had to: there he was, in the cells.

He got a message that his wife didn't want him back, and that she would be taking legal advice. He wasn't surprised given what he had been told, and what had been happening in recent months, the rows, the threats. He was sad, but he wasn't surprised. Felt he deserved it. He phoned in to work to say he was unwell, and would be off the day, hoped to be back on Friday. They wanted to know why he hadn't come in the previous day. He told them he had had some problems at home. His manager wanted to see him when he got in on Friday.

He then called one of his mates, Andy, to see if he could put him up in his flat for a few nights while he got his head straight. 'Wife's thrown me out, arrested, night in the cells, manager on my back at work, what a bloody awful night.' 'Sounds like you've been through it, mate,' was Andy's response. 'Sure you can stay round here. I'll be in the pub at lunchtime. Come and pick up a key.' The next week he drank heavily with Andy in the evenings. He hadn't bothered to go for the counselling. What was the point? He didn't really care. But he was beginning to miss his children. It built up and it was the day after he had missed his counselling appointment that he realised he couldn't go on like this. He phoned the counselling service and apologised. Alan wasn't there, but they took the message and said that a new appointment had been posted to him. He explained the situation and they gave him the appointment time over the phone. He had then spent the next few days trying to cut back a bit.

Wednesday morning, 1 November

Dave arrived on time, looking a bit worse for wear.

'Hi Dave, sorry not see you last week. I got your message. Glad you made it today. Looks like you've been through a lot.'

'Yeah. I need to talk. I need to make sense of things. It's all too much. Everything's gone wrong.'

'So you are feeling overwhelmed by what's been happening.'

'Yeah.' Dave told Alan about what had happened, and how he had ended up living with Andy for a few days. 'I don't know what triggered that drinking after I saw you, but one minute I was sitting in the park thinking, the next minute I was in the pub, and then I lost it. Don't remember what happened after about mid-afternoon. I think I went into blackout. Came out of it in the cells. Didn't know how I'd got there or what had happened. The police told me.'

> Alcohol blackouts are a common effect of seriously heavy drinking over a period of time. The drinker lives a period of life but the memories aren't stored, or at least, they can't be accessed later when the person comes out of blackout with no knowledge of what they have done or where they have been during the period of blackout. Scary stuff, can cause people to become highly anxious, even agoraphobic, fearful of whom they might meet because of not knowing what they had been doing.

'Scary. Must have been completely disorientated,' Alan responded, sensing just how frightening it must have been for Dave from his words and the way he had spoken them.

'Hadn't a clue what had been going on. I must have really hit the bottle to get like that. I've since found out that I went on from lagers to spirits, must have really tanked myself up. That's unusual for me. What I can't understand is why I went from the park to the pub, and it seems so quickly. One minute I must have been thinking about things, and I can remember sitting in the park, and then I was in the pub, and then I was in the cells. Why did I drink so heavily? I don't normally drink like that, and not all through the afternoon and evening.'

'So it was a really different drinking experience to what you are used to?' Alan sensed Dave's need to try and make sense of what had happened. It certainly sounded as though Dave had flipped into a state of mind with strong drinking associations. Anyway, now wasn't the time to theorise, stay with Dave as he goes over it. 'Yeah, it was so intense. It was the speed. It was almost as if I was another person, which sounds daft. But as though something took me over. I have never felt such an intense urge to drink like that.'

'The urge was incredibly intense. Sounds almost irresistible?'

'Yeah. Well, I wasn't resisting. I don't remember thinking of resisting. Get a drink, that was all I was thinking. And I did.'

'Get a drink, get a drink.'

'Yeah.' Dave lapsed into silence. 'Why?'

'Why?' There wasn't much else to be said and the 'why' remained unanswered.

'What the hell got into me?'

Alan could feel the temptation in the back of his mind to try and answer Dave's questions, but he knew instinctively that he must let Dave seek his own answers. He was there to support him. This was a key aspect to the person-centred approach, allowing the client to make their own way towards their answers. Coming in too quickly with suggestions, or trying to help the client make sense of something or draw connections and conclusions from the counsellor's perspective could only serve to confuse the client, and had the potential to damage a client's sometimes fragile attempts to begin to connect tentatively with, and trust, their own judgements.

'I really want to remember what was going on,' Dave finally said, his voice somewhat subdued, emphasising the *what was going on.*

'Yeah, sounds so important for you to remember what was going on, what was happening for you before and during that drinking episode.'

Alan suddenly felt loneliness seep over him and it wouldn't go away. He could feel for Dave in his lonely struggle to make sense of what had happened, and he felt loneliness in himself. It persisted. Should he voice it? Was it relevant? He knew that persistent feelings usually were important, but he was wary because he knew that he had his own stuff around loneliness and didn't want to project that into the situation. But it wouldn't go away. He knew from his training that it was often helpful to voice persistent feelings, but were they appropriate? It was no good. They *were* getting in the way. He had to say something.

'Dave, I don't know if this is relevant, but I am sitting here with a profound sense of loneliness. Does that have any bearing on anything?'

Dave looked up, then closed his eyes and took in a deep breath. He opened them slowly, aware of the goose bumps going up his face and down his back and arms. 'How did you know? That's it. Yeah. I can feel it and I can remember sitting there in the park. And yes, I was feeling so alone with it all. So alone. Then I have images of being in the pub, and then it was the cells. Oh God, I can feel that loneliness creeping up on me now.'

'That part of you that feels so alone is really present for you again.'

'It's awful. I feel like I'm shrivelling up into nothingness, and I feel a cold sensation all over my body. I'm shaking. Fucking hell. What's happening to me?'

Alan felt concerned – Dave wasn't withdrawing from alcohol, was he? 'Have you had a drink today, Dave? Wondering if you're withdrawing.'

'No, but I had a session last night, a little less than I had been. It doesn't feel like I'm needing a drink, just feel so small, so small.'

'So small . . . ,' Alan said it quite softly, it seemed as though maybe Dave was connecting with some deeper loneliness from his past perhaps.

Dave breathed deeply a few times, closed his eyes and tried to regain his bearings. The shaking had stopped but he still felt small in a big scary world, not just small but very, very alone.

Alan watched Dave as he seemed to be retreating back into the chair. He felt his sense of perspective shifting. Alan often experienced this with clients in moments of deep contact. It was as though the size of the room changed and the sense of himself apart from Dave was dissolving. He had learned to stay with this. In the early days it had felt scary and he had found it hard. Now he was more open to the experience, and trusting of it as part of the process of connecting at depth. It seemed that when some really deep aspect of the client was touched and brought into the therapeutic relationship, all kinds of experiencing could become present. Not only did it have a spatial effect, Alan had also noticed that time seemed to be affected too, as though time ceased to be regular but stretched or contracted. Usually in such moments it seemed to stretch; so much could happen in what was a short space of time. It reminded him of Salvador Dali's wonderful sculptures of elastic time-pieces.

'So small . . . ,' Alan repeated, again softly, not wanting to disturb Dave but feeling he wanted to communicate his presence and his empathy for what was happening to Dave.

Dave was drawing his knees up, and was putting his arms around them, and beginning to rock gently to and fro. 'She doesn't love me,' Dave said it in a childlike whimper.

'She doesn't like Dave.'

'David.'

'She doesn't like David,' Alan said, switching to Dave's words.

'She never cuddles me. On my own. In my room. So lonely. So frightened.'

'David never gets cuddles.' Should I keep in third person or switch to second? Alan only had a second to make the decision. 'On your own, in your room, so lonely, so frightened.'

'So alone.' Dave lapsed into silence again, still holding his knees and rocking gently. He really has connected with a part of himself from a long way back, Alan thought.

'It's lonely in that room. How old are you?'

'Six, but I'll soon be seven. Another birthday. I hate birthdays. Other children have parties. I don't. It's so lonely in here, and cold.'

'Cold and alone.' Alan was totally absorbed on Dave now, he was experiencing nothing outside of the relationship, no thoughts or feelings or any sense of self distinct from the connection with Dave. He felt bathed in compassion for this little boy, all alone in his room, not having birthday parties. 'Help me.' Dave looked up, his eyes seemed to have altered. They were wide and pleading, and full of tears.

'What would you like me to do?' Alan asked gently, experiencing a powerful urge to reach out and touch Dave, yet finding himself remaining in his chair, only his heart reaching out.

'Tell me it's OK; tell me that I'm OK. Tell me I'll wake up and it will be a bad dream.'

'I think you are OK, David, you are having a bad experience and it will end.'

Dave sighed, taking a deep breath, and appeared to collapse even further back into his chair, his eyes closed. Minutes passed. Alan could feel a shift taking place again. The connection was moving and he was becoming more aware of the surroundings once more, and of his own distinctive self. He guessed this was happening for Dave as well.

Dave opened his eyes; he was still feeling tremendously lonely, and not at all sure what had just happened. He was sitting with his arms round his knees. He didn't remember being like that. He sat back up. He remembered feeling shaky and cold, then . . . well, nothing. No, no he could remember seeing his bedroom when he was a boy, the blue curtains and the Fred Flintstone poster on the wall. He hadn't thought about that in years. 'What happened?'

'Can you remember? It might be important for you to try and connect with what happened.'

'I could see my bedroom when I was a boy, the curtains, the Fred Flintstone poster at the foot of the bed. I remember feeling the loneliness, and I can still feel that, so vivid, like it had all just happened, was happening, is happening now. I don't remember saying anything, but I do have the image of the room. Did I say anything?'

'Well you seemed to get in touch with something deep within you, a strong sense of loneliness as you say. You said you were six, nearly seven, that 'she' didn't love you, that you didn't get cuddles and that you hated birthdays. You asked me to tell you if you were OK and that you would wake up and that it was a bad dream. I told you that you were OK, and that the experience would end. That was when you came out of it.'

'I don't remember . . . .' Dave was shaking his head, as if trying to clear it and get his bearings once more. 'Whatever happened?'

'Seems like you made a deep connection with a very lonely little boy.'

Dave let out a sigh and a long breath. 'I feel strangely calm, incredibly calm. I've never felt like this before in my life. It's like being drunk, no, it's not because I feel so aware, so clear.' He let out a deep breath again.

'Incredibly calm, so aware, so clear?'

'Yeah. What else did I say?'

'You insisted I call you David.'

Dave smiled, and he shook his head not so much in disbelief as amazement. 'You know, that's what my mother always called me. Well, most people did, except for the other children. They called me Dave, well my friends did. I didn't have many friends. Haven't been called David in years.'

'Was your mother the 'she' who didn't cuddle you?' Alan asked, wondering if it was appropriate to ask but feeling it made sense to explore what Dave had said whilst the experience was still so close.

'Yes. Never cuddled me. I was a problem for her, got in the way. She brought me up on her own after my dad left when I was three. Hardly remember him. Saw the odd photo later but never had any contact with him.' Dave closed his eyes again and raised his hands to his face drawing them down over his mouth. He looked at Alan, shaking his head. 'I've never experienced anything like that. I feel I want to stay with it and I'm aware of the time and the need to get myself together and to leave. It feels so safe in here, but out there . . . I still feel like a little boy.'

'Still feel like a little boy.'

'Yeah.' Dave lapsed into silence and Alan was very aware of the time.

'Take your time; there's no rush. I want you to feel ready to go back out the door. You've had a really powerful experience. Want a cup of tea or some water?'

'Cup of tea would be good, one sugar.' Alan buzzed the intercom and the receptionist was asked to get a cup of tea, one sugar.

'So, what now?'

'Well, it seems that inside you is a very lonely part of yourself that goes back a long way. It is a part of you that when you connect with it you lose conscious touch with your day-to-day sense of self. You remember little of the experience in terms of what you said or felt, but only images from the past.' Alan felt it was OK to say this. He didn't feel he was saying anything that Dave had not already said or known.

'I used to spend so many hours looking at those walls, I'm not surprised.'

Alan felt that he needed to respond far more person-to-person than therapist-to client, as clearly Dave was preparing himself to head back out the door. The tea arrived.

'I thought I had something to think about when I left last time, but this is something else.'

'Yeah, a lot to think about. You did some thinking last time after the session?'

'Yeah, in the park, and that's when I . . . .' Dave went quiet.

'What is it, Dave?' Alan enquired.

'That's when I went so lonely, when I . . . you don't think I connected with, well, with whatever just happened?'

'Maybe.'

'But why did I drink? I didn't learn that when I was six.' Dave looked puzzled, he felt it. What the hell was going on? Why had he drunk?

'What feeling did you drink on Dave?'

'Being alone. Feeling lonely . . . feeling so, so lonely.'

'And then you drink?'

'Yeah, that's it. Lonely me drinks.'

Alan could sense what was going on. Dave had connected with a drinking config- uration within his self-structure, but now was not the time to start thinking about that. That's for reflection after the session, and supervision.

'You need to watch out for "lonely me" then.' That was a stupid thing to say, Alan thought immediately. Damn. OK, so *lonely me* may be causing problems, but like any other bit of you it needs to feel warmly accepted. 'No, not watch out for, perhaps get to understand and accept. After all, it is part of you.'

'Yeah. Hey, isn't this a bit weird?'

'It feels weird talking like this?'

'Well yes, and no. It makes so much sense. So there's a bit of me, "lonely me" let's say, that can trigger me into drinking, and really bingeing as well. I did drink differently on that loneliness.' Dave sat and thought about it for a moment. 'Loneliness, I've really got to watch that part of me. At least coming here means I'm not completely alone with it!' Dave smiled, but he knew it wasn't a very deep smile. He was worried about his 'lonely me' sense of self.

Alan saw the concern on Dave's face and responded to it. 'Concerned?'

'Yeah.' Dave took a deep breath and said, 'OK, time to think about moving on.'

The session slowly came to an end. Dave said he had lost track of his drinking since the last session, and wanted to try and keep tabs on it during the next week. He asked for some more drinking diary sheets. He hadn't a clue where the others had gone. Alan gave him a couple. They made an appointment for next week.

Alan ended by mentioning to Dave that if he felt he needed it Dave could call him at the counselling centre. He felt he wanted to extend his acceptance of Dave a little more, and he was concerned. Dave was clearly in a fragile place with a lot of uncertainties in his life at the moment. And yet he also felt he trusted Dave, or at least that 'actualising tendency' Rogers wrote of as 'the directional trend which is evident in all organic and human life – the urge to expand, extend, develop, mature – the tendency to express and activate all the capacities of the organism, or the self' (Rogers, 1961, p.351). 'The only function of the therapist is to facilitate the client's actualising process' (Bozarth, 1998, p.6). Bozarth had also included a reference to something Rogers had written in 1963, where the actualising tendency is described as a 'directional growth directed process that includes movement towards realisation, fulfilment and perfection of inherent capabilities and potentialities of the individual' (Bozarth, 1998, p.6). He, Alan, deeply trusted that. If he could provide the right therapeutic relationship and environment, he knew this tendency would nudge Dave towards his potential, and part of that process would be resolving his 'lonely me' configuration.

Summary

A powerful session in which Dave connects with a 'lonely me' configuration of self that is associated with his alcohol use. He reconnects with himself as a small boy and brings his experience into the session. Alan allows Dave to do this, adjusting his tone to take into account the shift that Dave has experienced. Spatial and time distortions occur as these deep memories are relived. Dave's 'lonely me' sense of self is fragile and vulnerable but he now has valuable self-insight into what lies behind his drinking.

Points for discussion

- What thoughts and feelings does this chapter bring to the surface for you?
- Alan introduced the theme of loneliness out of his own experiencing. How do you judge whether it is therapeutically helpful and valid to voice such experiences within a session?
- At one point Alan explains to Dave what has happened to him. Is this appropriate?
- What do you understand by the term 'drinking configuration' and how might this develop?
- Alan reflects on the notion of an 'actualising tendency'. What does this mean to you?

Wider focus

- When working with people with drinking problems it is important to think about what may lie beneath the drinking behaviour. It is frequently some hurt, trauma or unresolved loss.
- Many drinkers have drinking configurations, and thinking in this way can help to make sense of what is occurring for people.
- Working at depth with clients, particularly when they regress, is specialist work. Where this occurs, or is likely to occur, and you are not adequately trained and supervised for this work, refer to a counsellor or therapist who is.

Friday afternoon, 3 November

'Jan, I've got to spend time exploring what's happening with Dave. So much has occurred since I last saw you and the last session was so powerful. He really connected with some deep, childhood feelings and I was so drained after that session.' Alan knew he had to focus on Dave. He was still so aware of the last session. It was incredibly vivid and he had struggled to hold it until supervision.

'What's been happening then, Alan? I can't help noticing that you look pretty tense.'

'Well, Dave has been for two more sessions, and the middle one he didn't attend. After the first session he told me he went for a couple of beers, phoned in and didn't go to work that afternoon. Told me he was feeling quite bad after the session, had a row with his wife and spent most evenings the following week in the pub. I think he had had a can before coming to the second session, although he denied it. He told me that he had been in two minds about coming. But he made it, and described his drinking pattern – evenings in the pub, sometimes cans at home, a few pints in the pub at lunchtimes. Seemed to be getting up to around the 20 or so units a day mark. I was concerned, wondering if he was dependent.'

Jan was very aware that Alan was just repeating the history and she sensed that this was leading to something far more emotional. She did not interrupt but let him continue with his description.

Alan carried on, 'He seemed motivated to want to change, aware of what he had to lose. That second session, though, seemed to have stirred up a lot of stuff. He began to face up to the fact that he had a drink problem, and he was really struggling to accept this. He wanted to know what I thought, and I told him that I did think he had a problem. It didn't seem right to just reflect back his wanting to know if he had a problem. And there was a point where he was saying he needed time to be on his own to think about it, and he became very silent after saying that. I didn't make much of it at the time – it really didn't stick with me – for he then moved on to talk about how could he tell people and what he should do.'

'So you sensed that silence. It obviously made an impression because you have remembered it but didn't respond to it at the time.'

'No. And I now really wonder whether I should and why I didn't.'

'Why you didn't respond to the silence?'

'It was fairly short and I suppose whilst it didn't make a great impression at the time, after the last session he attended it has taken on a fresh poignancy.'

'So what happened in the last session?' Jan asked.

'Well, he really did touch into the loneliness in himself. By the way, he didn't attend the appointment in between those two sessions. He had drunk heavily after the second session and ended up having a night in the police cells. He's now staying with a friend. His wife's told him she doesn't want him back. The whole chain of events seemed to have been triggered by that second session. He said he was sitting in the park thinking about things, and on his way back to work he had suddenly started feeling very anxious and had gone into the pub for a drink. Anyway, he got into this issue of feeling lonely about his drinking and having to face it, and then he flipped into himself as a six-year-old, on his own, in his room, feeling very lonely. Told me his mother never cuddled him, referring to her as 'she', and that his father had left when he was three. He became that six-year-old, he sat there hugging his knees to his chest, and he visibly went small. I felt an incredible connection to him. There was some spatial distortion in the room and I was, well, it was one of those moments I can never find the words for. Barriers dissolved, *I-thou* went out the window, we were connected, and to this six-year-old boy.'

'How were you feeling and what thoughts were going through your mind?' Jan didn't want to respond only by focusing on feelings; she knew that thoughts were important too.

'I remember feeling what I can only describe as compassion, my heart just went out to this little boy, particularly when he said, 'help me'. I just felt such compassion.' Alan could feel the tears welling up in his own eyes and a burning lump in his throat. 'It really got to me, and it still is.' Alan sat allowing the tears to flow for a minute or so, pleased to have such a safe and supportive space to allow himself to be his feelings. 'Told me he never got cuddles. How can anyone go through childhood like that?'

Jan was wondering whether Alan's reaction was an instinctive human reaction to what he had experienced with Dave, or whether it was touching into something Alan had also experienced. She felt she had to ask this as she had to consider the well-being of the client. If Alan had had a similar experience, he might need to do some therapeutic work on himself to be able to engage effectively with Dave at this kind of psychological depth. Working in this way with clients was powerful, and unresolved issues could become exacerbated with the therapist losing their ability to maintain congruence and their role as counsellor.

'Did you get cuddles as a child, Alan?' she asked gently, aware that this was a sensitive area and was uncertain how Alan would respond.

'Yes, I did. My mother was very tactile, and yeah, I did get hugs and cuddles. Part of my family's way of being. I guess it makes me so aware of what Dave missed.' Alan's voice became stronger as he said it.

'Sounds like there's some anger there as well, Alan. You've got some strong feeling about this.' Jan could feel the atmosphere change. Alan was frowning and staring ahead of himself, and certainly looking angry.

'I mean, for Christ's sake, a six-year-old boy on his own, in a cold room, he said he was cold and lonely, I mean, that's emotional neglect. Parents should. . . . Oh shit!' Alan stopped speaking and his eyes watered again. He put his head in his hands and took a deep breath. Jan waited, she knew Alan well enough to know he could be trusted with his own process and to say what he needed to say when he needed to say it. 'Shit!' The word exploded from Alan's mouth again, he rubbed his eyes and looked up at Jan. 'Since my relationship break-up last year I only see my daughter a couple of times a week at most, and I miss hugging her. Always used to hug her in the mornings, last thing at night, and any times in between if she was upset, or anything. Oh hell, that's why I'm angry at Dave's mother. I'm also angry and frustrated myself that I can't give my daughter the hugs she needs.'

'You really miss that contact with her.' Jan was aware that this was straying into personal stuff, but it was relevant to the work with this client and had to be addressed.

'Yeah, hardest part of it all. OK, I know it's around now. I know I need to be aware of it and to watch my reactions. I don't want to stop being me with the client, but I don't want my issues to start becoming overly present in the relationship with Dave. I'm in fortnightly therapy. I'll take it back there. I thought I'd worked it through, but I guess you never really do. Dave has triggered me and I need to go and look at this again. I'm still carrying some pretty raw feelings, aren't I? I'll talk about this to my therapist. That feels the appropriate place to take it now that it has come clear. I just hadn't made the connection until just now. All I knew was that I had such a strong feeling reaction for Dave as that little boy. Is that OK? There are other aspects of working with Dave I want to explore which I think are more appropriate for here.'

'Sure you are ready to move on? Just want to check because you did experience a strong reaction.'

'Yes, I can see what's happening for me. Dave really has come along with some issues to press my buttons. I know we have talked about it before, but I do wonder about how clients seem to arrive with issues which provoke us to deal with aspects of our own stuff, even stuff we thought we had dealt with! I wonder sometimes, who's helping who!'

'It's not as simple as a client coming with a problem and a therapist helping them sort it out, is it?' Jan responded, aware that she was restraining a smile. She gave in.

'You can smile, yeah, I know. I guess it's the approach. In trying to apply person-centred principles I really want to bring my whole self into the therapeutic relationship with Dave so that I am fully available to the whole of him, or as much of himself that he feels able to bring into the session. It would be easier if we had a much more detached approach, but then, it wouldn't be person-centred, would it? The power of creating a therapeutic relationship is so overlooked I think sometimes by approaches that get all caught up in techniques and lose sight of that basic factor: relationship. Oops, slipped on to my soap-box there.'

'Don't apologise to me, Alan. I appreciate the passion you have for the approach and the depth of caring you offer to your clients. It's precious.'

'Yeah, it is.' Alan sat silently for a few moments, being with just how important this approach was for him. 'OK, I want to talk through with you what was in my mind when Dave was talking as himself as a six-year-old and expressing his deep loneliness. By the way, he referred to himself then as David – what he was called at that age. It struck me during the session, and I put it to one side to reflect on later and to discuss here, that Dave was showing me a "configuration of self", you know, like Mearns has written about (Mearns, 1998, 1999). And I don't want to get into sounding like I am diagnosing here, but I think this "lonely me" is a "drinking configuration" (Bryant-Jefferies, 2001). I think his sense of profound loneliness is a major trigger for drinking. Certainly, in the instance after the second counselling session this feeling seemed to have played a major part in triggering Dave into drinking heavily, which led to all the problems.'

Jan was familiar with this idea, and it certainly sounded plausible. As people develop they create within their self-structure discreet identities with atten-dant sets of associated feelings, or is it the other way round, she wondered, identity forming in response to feelings? Anyway, the idea is that if the child, or even adult, experiences enough reinforcement of a particular set of feelings, then they become part of that person's sense of self, and because they arise frequently they have to be made acceptable. Hence they become identified with. However, the child or adult then chooses certain behaviours in response to those feelings. If they are uncomfortable then they may choose some response that helps to ease the discomfort. One use of alcohol is to dull discomfort. Now, she'd read something in an autobiography recently, yes, it was in *Drinking: a love story*, the idea of equations that people with alcohol problems create in their minds, in this case 'Discom-fort + alcohol = no discomfort' (Knapp, 1996, p.61). Self-transformation, with alcohol the magic wand.

'So, you think Dave has a "lonely me" drinking configuration, and he's drinking on it. Well, maybe one of the reasons he is drinking is to ease the discomfort.'

'I think so. I'm sure he has other drinking triggers, but this one certainly came through this time, and he noted his intensity of drinking, which was unusual. So maybe this drinking configuration has to be set against more of a habit pat-tern as well.'

'And, of course, that may be linked into configurations as well. He drinks with his mates in the pub, right? So his social identity and the feelings associated with that are also a factor.'

'Yeah, and I wonder how much of the rowing at home could be orchestrated to give him a reason to go to the pub.' Alan was aware that he hadn't really thought this through before now in relation to Dave.

'OK, let's not let the speculation run away with us, but we can be aware that we could have multi-configurational drinking here with Dave. You'll just have to see what else emerges as he talks about the feelings associated with drinking and, of course, not drinking.' Jan was suddenly aware that she had cut across Alan there, and wondered why. She decided to mention it. 'I think something just happened for me there. Somehow I didn't respond to your idea that the pub drinking could be orchestrated by his wife to get him to go down the pub.'

Alan felt bemused. That wasn't what he had meant. 'No, what I meant was that Dave was orchestrating the rows.'

Jan had genuinely heard something different and clearly had missed the point completely, or was she hearing something relevant but it just hadn't been said by Alan? 'Alan, I realise I attached a very different meaning to what you said and I do not know why. I need to take this to my own supervision and check it out. It has clearly stopped me hearing you accurately. Apologies for that.'

Supervisors need supervision as well. They can find themselves reacting in ways that are disconnected to what is being present, and the need to talk it through and make sense of their reaction is a professional response. Sometimes it can be talked through more fully within the supervision session in which it occurs as it can have relevance, even though it may not seem to have.

'That's OK. But it may have some truth to it as well. I guess we don't know enough about Dave's wife to know yet. But it is possible. I know this because I've seen it happen before. It could be that she triggers the rows to get him to choose to go down the pub. Why this may be, I don't know, but there could be something from her past here as well. What I need to do is to keep my thoughts and feelings open to whatever comes along.'

'Anything is possible. You say she was going to come to a counselling session?'

'Well, we discussed this and Dave was going to talk to her about it. Of course, as he isn't under the same roof with her now, that seems somewhat unlikely.'

'Would you see them together if an opportunity arose, having already begun work with Dave and clearly having quite quickly created a relationship which allows him to bring quite deep psychological content into the session?'

'I guess things have changed since we first talked about it. Maybe it would be good to go over this now, just in case it comes up again. I'm sure that if Dave does get back with his wife, it will come up. There always seems to be more to it when alcohol affects relationships. I wonder what Dave's wife's background is. He hasn't said anything.'

'We'll have to wait for that. OK. So, Dave says to you, "How about bringing my wife to the next session?" How are you going to respond, and what issues are going to be around?'

'Well, I already have a relationship forming with Dave, and will need to ensure that I maintain confidentiality with regard to that relationship.'

'OK, that seems pretty important. You'll be sitting there knowing things that his wife does not know. You may even hear her say things that are different to what Dave has said.'

'True, although Dave has said very little about his marriage yet. This could of course change before a possible joint session.'

'You say a "joint session". How joint do you mean?'

'Well, I wouldn't see it as couple counselling, although I am also open to discuss this with Dave and with his wife. But I generally offer a joint session for both partners as a kind of information exchange, to help the partner get an understanding of what is going on, or what alcohol problems mean and how difficult they can be to resolve. Also to discuss what the partner can offer, and in this obviously I would imagine there would be input from Dave.'

'OK, so not couple counselling as such. The deeper work will remain with Dave, and the session with both of them would probably be about information exchange. What if they wanted actual therapeutic couple counselling?' Jan knew she was being a bit of a devil's advocate, but she wanted to be sure Alan had thought it through. She felt sure he had, but with issues around a bit close to home for Alan, she felt this was professionally important.

'No, I don't think I would offer this. I sense already that Dave needs his own space to work at depth. I think if they want to work on issues in their relationship over a period of time they would need to seek a couples counsellor. I feel clear on that.'

'OK, so an information session with them both is acceptable but therapeutic counselling for them both you would not offer. Dave is your client and you would see your allegiance to him.'

'Yeah, it's a professional commitment. But we'll see, it may never happen. But then, the fact that we have dwelt on it today kind of leaves me thinking it is going to come up. It is strange how things that get talked about in supervision do end up being relevant. But we will see.'

When working with a client, the possibility of seeing them with their partner always has to be thought through carefully. In this case, Alan is clear that it will be an information session. However, sometimes things happen in the moment that takes an information session into a more therapeutic encounter. Dave is in a fragile state and his loneliness has become much closer to the surface of his experiencing. It may come through again in the couple session and Alan will need to feel confident to respond to this in a way that is supportive of Dave and yet attends to the needs of his wife, who could be quite shocked.

'OK. Anything more you want to talk through about Dave? I'm just checking with myself too to see if there is anything left with me that I want to mention. I see myself as being here to recognise content and process that passes you by. Let's just take a couple of minutes to reflect quietly on where we both are with the work you are doing with Dave.'

As Alan sat there quietly taking stock of himself and allowing his awareness to be with both himself and the relationship he had with Dave, he felt himself become very calm. His mind went back to the compassion he had felt. It was compassion. He had experienced an emotional reaction, but somehow this was coming from somewhere deeper. He felt an inner assurance that all would be well, though he couldn't explain what would be well or how it would all work out. It felt . . . , the only word he could think of was *spiritual*.

Jan was reflecting on how she had felt earlier in the session when Alan first began talking and how she felt in the present moment. She too had a feeling of calm assurance and she was mindful as well that Dave was probably not going to find change easy given his alcohol use, the depth of his loneliness and the possibility of other complicating factors that had yet to emerge. But she knew that the process of growth was trustworthy, and that within himself Dave had an instinctive urge to grow towards realising fuller potential of himself as a person. And Alan had clearly established a climate of trust. There was so much vulnerability being made present by Dave within the sessions. Alan was doing good work here. Dave was bringing more and more of himself into the sessions, offering himself the opportunity, through his relationship with Alan, to explore and redefine himself as a person, and hopefully resolve the knots of uncomfortable feeling that had become very much lodged within his personality from those early life experiences.

Jan was aware of how much she really enjoyed giving supervision, and feeling able to help colleagues help others. It felt like a kind of 'therapeutic chain of service' and it felt good to be part of it. She knew she had to be there for Alan on his journey with this client, and was glad he was in personal therapy. Yet she knew, too, her first allegiance was with Dave. Always seemed funny that the person she was there to protect and to be mindful of was the person she never met. That was one of the quirks of professional counselling. But she didn't need to meet Alan's clients since, in a very real way, she did meet them in supervision. In fact, she was concerned when a supervisee could not bring a client clearly into the room. It generally meant that there was not a good connection with the client, or something was being hidden or not spoken about that needed to be made visible.

Alan spoke first. 'Just struck me what a sense of spirituality there is with Dave somehow, something to do with the depth of connection we had for a while. I guess I'm now wondering how he experienced it, and how he is processing it between sessions. We do tend to think of our one hour with clients as being so important, which it often is, but they then have 167 hours to be on their own with whatever has taken place in that one hour. Takes a lot of courage . . . or desperation, to come into counselling.'

'How do you feel Dave will be this week?'

'I don't know. The optimist in me feels he will be OK, yet I appreciate how difficult it is for him, how so many areas of his life are uncertain at the moment. But I do have this sense that all will be well, eventually.'

'My thoughts ended up with how sometimes supervisees do not voice aspects of their experience with clients, and how it can leave me feeling disconnected. However, I feel connected to Dave, through you, and I want to say that I appreciate your openness about him and your ability and willingness to bring your feelings, reactions and thoughts into the room here and into our relationship.'

> Jan felt it important to give positive feedback to supervisees when she felt it. Supervision was, after all, collaborative, and not some kind of 'teacher–pupil' relationship.

'Thanks.' Alan grinned. 'Actually, I didn't have a lot of choice in the matter today. Those feelings and reactions in me were so present that they just had to be made visible to you. Besides, what's the point of supervision if you don't use it? Anyway, I feel you would have picked up on any incongruence I may have had between what I was experiencing and what I was saying.'

'I hope so too. Not everyone understands it that way. People can be quite defensive, particularly when they start with a new supervisor. It is important for me to make it collaborative. We sit here in effect with the client between us trying to figure out our reactions, their reactions and generally what is going on. Helps us all to get clear, and for you to be less cluttered when you next meet them, and sometimes have ideas about what to look out for or be particularly sensitive towards.'

'Yeah, well, I'm seeing Dave next Wednesday and we'll see what he brings. He's gone off with a drinking diary again, be interesting to see if he fills it in and, if so, what this week has been like. Thanks for all that, Jan, I feel I have unloaded and clarified, I feel freer and ready to move on.'

'OK, who else do you want to talk about today . . . ?'

So the supervision session ended insofar as Dave was concerned. Meanwhile, Dave was getting back with his wife, and they were going to be talking soon about coming to a future counselling session with Alan.

Summary

Alan describes the previous session and Jan picks up on Alan's strong sensitivity to Dave's experience as a child. She raises it as it is intense and it leads to Alan realising that it has been too close to his own recent experience, which he has decided to look at in his own personal therapy. Jan also mis-hears something Alan says and realises she must take this to her own supervision. Together they reflect on Dave's experience from the theoretic standpoint of 'drinking configurations'. Alan reflects on his sense of connection with Dave as having some spiritual quality whilst Jan reflects on what Alan is achieving with Dave and the importance of supervision as a collaborative process.

Points for discussion

- How can Alan ensure that his own feelings do not obstruct his ability to empathise with Dave's inner world?
- How has this supervision session informed Alan's practice and deepened his understanding of Dave?
- Does the concept of 'drinking configurations' seem clearer to you?
- What is the advantage of supervision that allows you to explore process and personal experience?
- Should counsellors be in personal therapy all the time or only when they feel they need it?
- What is the benefit to supervisors, their supervisees and their clients of having supervision of their practice?

Wider focus

All professionals working with people can benefit from supervision, and so can their clients. Issues can be touched on that trigger off strong reactions that are not fully appreciated for what they are at the time, leading to unhelpful and confusing reaction to clients. At the least, a period of personal therapy to explore attitudes towards a given client group is likely to be helpful and raise awareness of associated issues and attitudes that could obstruct the creation of helpful relationships.

Wednesday morning, 8 November

Dave arrived on time and came into the room with his drinking diary in his hand. He looked more positive and certainly in a better state than he had for the last counselling session, or so Alan thought as he watched him come in. He thought he would mention it as it had struck him so forcibly.

'You are looking well, Dave, looking quite positive in fact.'

'I am. Things have taken a positive turn this week and I am feeling good. There's still a long way to go but I feel as if I have made a start.'

'So feeling good, feeling positive, and you feel you have made a start on this long journey.' That felt a bit wordy, thought Alan, but it seemed to sum it all up.

'Yes, I'm back at home.'

'You look almost surprised in saying that, and I think I am feeling surprised as well.' Alan was being congruent to what he read into Dave's expression and his own reaction.

'Well, my wife called me at work after I'd seen you last week My son Ian wasn't well. He'd been playing up wanting to know where daddy was. Linda called me because she didn't know what to do. It got rather emotional and I said I'd call round later, which I did. And we talked, and got emotional again, and I said I was sorry and that I had realised how much I was losing, and that I didn't want to lose everything; that I loved her and that I really wanted to do something about my drinking. She said she was sorry she had said she didn't want me back, but didn't know what else to do. Everything had seemed so out of control, she was afraid, and she was afraid for the children.'

'Afraid for the children.' Dave seemed in full flow. Alan didn't want to disturb this, didn't see any need to use lots of words to empathise with all that had been said.

The hardest empathic responses are often the brief ones. The one-word response, perhaps the last word in a paragraph, can be enough for the client to feel listened to without interrupting their flow. Counsellors do not have to show empathy to every detail. Allow the client to flow. If they feel something has not been heard they will soon repeat it. It was Horace who said that 'it is when I struggle to be brief that I become obscure'.

'Yeah, that really got to me. I mean, I couldn't, wouldn't want to do anything to hurt them.'

'Couldn't, wouldn't want to hurt your children.' Alan allowed his voice to drop.

'I love them, man. I missed them so much. Ian's nine, the oldest, and my two daughters, Emily and Jane, are six and four. It's so good to be back home again.'

'So good to be with them again.'

'Oh yeah. Hey, and I've really tried with the drinking. I really have. This week I'm off the lunchtime beers. Monday I stayed in the office and had sandwiches and read the paper. It wasn't easy, but I was determined. I've had a taste of what I was losing. Yesterday I went for a walk, over the park. Thank goodness it was sunny. I think that helped. And I'm drinking more non-alcoholic drinks. Living on tea at work, having a bit more sugar in it for some reason, but it's OK.'

'You sound determined. Sugar could be to compensate for the sugar from the alcohol. Not unusual for people to compensate with extra sweet things. Just need to be sure it doesn't get out of control.' Alan felt it was important to say this, so Dave had an understanding that this was normal, but at the same time it did need to be kept an eye on.

People can develop a sugar addiction coming off alcohol. It is probably better for the client to compensate for the sugar they are no longer getting from the alcohol with carbohydrates. However, carrying sugary sweets to eat can stave off a craving for alcohol.

'Yeah, I am determined. Been shaky, sweaty at night, not sleeping too well, but I'm OK. I'm going to get over this, I bloody well am, I have to.'

'Mhmmm. Good for you. I hear your determination.' Alan then added, ' "Bloody well have to" seems to sum it up.'

'Too much to lose. I've got to get on top of it. It's good to feel I've got control over the lunch times.' Dave did feel good, felt he had achieved a great deal. So did Alan, although Alan was also aware of his wondering about the evening drinking. Should he raise it, or let Dave keep his focus on lunch times and what he had achieved? He decided to leave Dave with his focus, accepting Dave knew what he wanted to talk about. If nothing was said then he would raise it later.

'Yeah, and I've made changes in the evening as well.'

'I was wondering about the evening drinking. Where's that at?' Alan replied, pleased to hear that changes had happened there as well. Maybe Dave isn't as dependent as he had thought.

'Well, I moved back home Saturday morning. Since then I've stayed in during the evenings. I've still had some cans. I've kept a record here on the diary.' Dave passed the sheet over to Alan to look at. Four cans on Saturday, two Sunday lunchtime, six more Sunday evening, six Monday evening and six Tuesday evening. He noted that it was 5% lager, same brand. So running at about six cans a day, about 13 units by his reckoning. If Dave could hold it at that he would have taken a big step away from what had felt like alcohol dependence when he described the drinking pattern in that second session. Thirteen units a day meant that he had 13 hours of alcohol in his body, which meant 11 hours alcohol-free. His body needed time to adjust to this. However, Alan felt he should also check with Dave what reactions he had had to cutting back.

'So, sounds very positive, any other reactions apart from sweating, sleep disturbance and feeling shaky?'

'No, well, a little on edge at times, but I'm determined. Starting to try and eat a little more. My appetite had gone, but I'm beginning to eat again in the evenings. Don't have anything in the morning, just tea before going to work. Never did eat breakfasts.'

'So, appetite returning a little, drinking lots of non-alcoholic liquid, mainly tea, a few symptoms of withdrawal but nothing too serious by the sound of it. And you're determined.'

'Yeah. Also been talking it through with Linda. She has agreed to come to a counselling session here. Is that OK? She wants to talk to you. I think she's concerned that it will all go wrong again and is wondering what she can do to help. Her father had an alcohol problem, I know that, and I think, well, she wants to have a chat with you. So can she come along with me next time?'

Alan was pleased he had talked this through in supervision. Had it been a premonition! 'Fine, Dave, and I want you to know that you are still my client here and I would regard Linda coming as being an opportunity for information exchange. I would want to maintain confidentiality in terms of what you have told me. I leave it for you to tell her what you want her to know about what we have talked about in the sessions, and maybe what we'll talk about today.'

'That's fine, but can we make the next session slightly earlier, to fit in with Jane being at the nursery. Linda usually collects her at 12.00.'

'No problem. We can go for 10.00 am instead of 11.00 am. Will that be OK?'

'Yeah, thanks. She drops Jane off at 9.30 am, so that will work out well.'

'OK, so we have a little over 40 minutes left. What do you want to focus on today?'

'I'm not sure. So much going on at the moment. I guess my real concern is around how to make sure I keep in control, and what else I may need to do.' Whilst Dave sort of felt confident, he also knew that it hadn't been easy not to drink at lunch times. Monday had really not been easy. He'd kept looking at the clock on the wall opposite his desk. That's why he went out on Tuesday, stop him sitting there looking at the clock. Mind you, he kept looking at his watch, but it felt different being out the office. Yet he knew he couldn't go to the park every day. Hell, it was November, and whilst the weather seemed milder these days in the winter, he really had to have some other ideas for keeping away from the pub. He'd told his colleagues at work that he had been told by his GP to cut back, and after all the problems he had just had he was trying to follow that advice. Some had seemed supportive, some hadn't, trying to convince him it was up to him what he wanted to do, not to listen to what people told him. Few drinks didn't hurt. Well, a few weeks back Dave would have agreed, but now he wasn't so sure. He was determined to get control of his alcohol use and get his life back together at home.

'So, how to keep control and what else you might need to do as part of this change.' Alan felt he should convey empathy for what Dave was wanting, leaving the direction to Dave.

Alan firmly believed that the client can be trusted to know best – another key aspect of the person-centred approach. Rogers had himself written that 'the basic nature of the human being, when functioning freely, is constructive and trustworthy' (Rogers, 1961, p.194). The problem arises, however, when alcohol is a factor because it could be argued that heavy alcohol use disrupts the drinker's ability to function freely. Free functioning is linked to congruence. However, it has been argued that alcohol intake disrupts congruent experiencing (Bryant-Jefferies, 2001). In Alan's view, Dave was not alcohol-affected in this session and was therefore more likely to be realistic about his options and his goals.

'Yeah. The diary was good. Made me think about what I was doing,' was Dave's response. Alan noted that Dave had more to say about the diary before moving on, so he was pleased he hadn't directed him straight into planning. 'I hadn't really thought too much about how I felt before and after drinking, and certainly not about how much I was spending. And I've only been drinking cans from the off-licence. I was getting through so much more with the pub drinking.'

'Made you think, then?' Alan replied, again wanting to keep the focus open.

'Sure. I could see that the drinking really was linked to feeling on edge. It wasn't that I was exactly gagging for a pint, though it was a bit like that on the Monday lunch time at work, but it was as though all I could think of was having a drink. Couldn't focus on what I was doing – well, I was watching the TV, but my attention kept switching to the idea of opening one of the cans.'

'So the start of the evening drinking was more about not being able to focus on much other that that idea of opening the first can, whereas the Monday lunch time was more of a "gagging for a pint",' Alan responded, aware that he was struggling to distinguish 'not being able to avoid thinking of opening a can' and 'gagging for a pint'. He held the thought for the moment.

'Couldn't settle. Take Saturday. I'd got in at 5.00 pm, been out with my son to the sports centre, and immediately my thought was on that first can.'

'First thought of the can when you got home.'

'Yes, well, no, not exactly. I was aware of wanting a can before I got home.'

'OK, so your thoughts were towards that can earlier. What kind of time had they kicked in?' Alan felt it was important to have some idea of timing to help see if there was a pattern.

'I suppose from around 4.00 pm I was thinking, soon be home and can have a can or two.'

'So it was holding your attention when you were with your son, "soon be home and can have a can or two".'

'Yes, wasn't too good, was it.'

'Wasn't too good?' Alan replied with a hint of questioning in his tone of voice.

'Well, I really don't want to be thinking of drinking.'

'So it seems that what you were doing was not a strong or appealing enough focus for you to keep your thoughts away from the idea of that can or two when you got home.'

'No.' Dave paused for a moment. He continued, 'That feels really uncomfortable. I was watching my son going through his judo routines. He's really into it. He was doing really well, but I drifted.' Dave looked glum.

'Leaves you with uncomfortable feelings, not being able to hold your focus on your son.'

'I mean, he's my son, I want to focus on him, not on a bloody can of lager.'

'Yes, your son is important to you, that's where you want your focus, not on "a bloody can of lager".' Alan emphasised these words that Dave had used, they had power and he wanted to show that he had heard them.

Dave sat in silence for a while. 'I really want to be there for him, you know, really be there, not with half of me thinking about having a drink. That's why I need help. I know I'm doing well, but I also know I'm on the edge here. It might not take much for me to slip back again. What do you think?'

Alan took a moment to be with his own thoughts and feelings and noted he also felt that Dave was on the edge, that it was early days and he really needed to work at maintaining what he had achieved so far. He voiced his thoughts, 'You want to be there for your son. You really do want to be there for him. You feel on edge and I sense this too, and that it wouldn't take much to trigger you into heavy drinking. It's about maintaining change, isn't it, and what you can do to try and ensure that you at least maintain your current drinking pattern.'

'I'd like to cut back more, but can't see it just at the moment. Do you think I'm going about this the right way?'

'So you're not too sure whether this is the best way forward. You want to cut back some more, but just now that seems a big step?' Alan again voiced his response somewhat as a question, wanting to check out he really was grasping Dave's dilemma.

'I guess I'm confused. I feel as if I have achieved change, and I am unsatisfied because I want to achieve more. But I'm also unhappy because I feel as though I can't push it too much.'

'Kind of feel you can walk but not ready to run, as it were?' Alan liked to use metaphors, and this did seem to sum up what he was hearing from Dave, but was it what Dave was trying to communicate?

'Yeah. Afraid I'll run back to the pub, or for another can or something. It's going to be one step at a time, isn't it?'

'One step at a time and your fear is that you'll not be able to maintain the change. So I guess we either focus here on the fear and what that is related to, or the kind of strategies to try and ensure you give yourself the best chance of maintaining change.'

Dave sat silently, and Alan was aware that he felt that Dave was more focused on the fear than on strategies. How he sensed this, he did not know, but this was counselling. Sometimes you felt things and did not know quite where they were coming from. He didn't like the idea that it was Dave passing it across to him in some way, rather more that something in him was experiencing fear for the kind of situation Dave was facing. Should he say something? He didn't want to direct Dave. Alan stayed silent for the moment.

When to speak and when to stay silent comes from experience and the ability to be in relationship to the client and empathic to their inner world. Sometimes it can feel like a dance, and in the same way that some steps are planned and some are more spontaneous, so it can be in the counselling relationship.

'What do you think?' Dave asked. 'I don't know which way to go with this.'

'I don't know what to think, but I am sitting here with a sense of the fear you have of lapsing back to your old drinking pattern.'

'Yeah, that's what's with me too. I don't want to mess up. I've been thrown out once. I don't want to go through that again. I couldn't face that. It's made me realise how lonely I'd be without my kids, and without my wife. They are so important to me. Without them, well it's just emptiness.'

'Emptiness,' Alan responded, nodding his head slightly and taking a deep breath and releasing it. The short empathic response was often more powerful than long reflections.

Alan smiled inwardly. How many times had he heard clients struggling with loneliness and emptiness – two very different things, although often used interchangeably. Loneliness was linked to not having people around. Emptiness went further and was often simply a void, no people, no hope, nothing.

Dave took a deep breath, and sat in silence. He was looking down again. 'Without them I can't see a future.' Another silence. 'I'm feeling really queasy inside, stomach churning again.' Dave took another deep breath and let it out slowly.

'Without them you can't see a future.'

Dave was quiet. Alan could sense Dave was heading back into that lonely place again. 'Just take it slowly, breathe slowly and deeply.' He was a little surprised how quickly Dave seemed to access this, yet he hadn't said anything about experiencing it before. Either he has been here in the past and not mentioned it, Alan thought, or it is really near the surface of his awareness. He kind of felt it was the latter, as if the time was right and Dave's own growth process was forcing him to face his 'lonely me' sense of self.

'It's like a pit, a deep, dark pit.'

'A deep, dark pit. You inside it?' Alan wasn't sure why he asked that, bit of an assumption.

'No, it's inside me.'

Oh well, thought Alan, it was an assumption. Might need to explore that one in supervision. Anyway, usually it doesn't matter if you miss the target sometimes. Clients are good at putting you right so long as your intention is to understand. So long as you don't make a habit of it ...

'It's like a dark hole inside myself, it feels ...,' Dave's sentence trailed off into silence. Alan waited. Nothing was said, minutes passed. Dave was sitting, his eyes open, still staring at the floor, his elbows on his knees. Alan wasn't sure whether to say something. He really wanted to let Dave know he was there. He was striving to be in touch with where Dave was, but he didn't want to disturb him. Perhaps Dave needed to sit in this experience. There was plenty of time to go in the session, time for Dave to continue and have time to reorient himself ready to go home. Hold on, Alan thought, I'm drifting. I need to be with Dave, not speculate about what comes later. What do I say? Focus him on the 'dark hole', or on the 'it feels'? Tell him I'm here if he needs me? No, that would risk shifting his focus out of himself.

Silences occur and the counsellor needs to feel able to sit with them. Clients can need silences to work in. Occasional, minimal comments from the counsellor can ensure the client knows they have a companion, but they need to be gentle, respectful of the silence. The counsellor can helpfully be empathic to the silent communication from the client, reflecting it back through their own observed silence.

Sometimes a silence feels very much like a working silence, the client is in process. At other times it can feel very stuck, or awkward. Where is the stuckness or awkwardness residing? In the client? In the counsellor? Or in both? It may then need voicing but with ownership. 'I'm not sure if this is how it is for you but this silence feels awkward.' It can be a new experience for someone to sit in silence with another and often new experiences bring anxiety. Or silences may have particular associations for the client, and for the counsellor.

'It feels ...,' Alan said softly, trying to float the words out as gently as he could, inviting Dave to respond if he wanted to.

Dave wasn't sure what he was feeling. He was actually numb, feeling psychologically and emotionally paralysed. Yet he wasn't thinking of those words. He was simply lost in ..., well, not in thought because he wasn't thinking. He was lost in the pit inside himself. But he wasn't thinking of a pit. He was just being, nothing going through his head, no feeling passing through him at all. He was just ... he just was. He couldn't move; he didn't want to move; he didn't have a concept of movement as he sat motionless, staring into space.

The silence continued and the minutes passed. Alan sought to reach into Dave's world. How could he communicate his presence? He did not feel a companion to

Dave at this moment. Dave seemed to be in a place in himself that Alan could not reach. All Dave was giving him was silence and stillness. This was what Alan offered back as he, too, sat motionless in silence, watching Dave and seeking to remain alert to anything Dave might wish to communicate. Sometimes empathic responses are not about the words, but how the therapist is with the client. Alan felt he was conveying empathy by respecting Dave's choice and right to be silent.

Dave drew in a deep breath and closed his eyes. He heard Alan take a deep breath too, and heard him say, 'If you want to stay in the silence, it's OK.' The emptiness was dissipating now, as if he, Dave, had pulled back from it, or had it pulled back from him? It was there, inside himself, but he was beside it now. He felt calm. It was the first thing he seemed to have felt for a long time. He still had his eyes closed. Slowly he opened them and focused on Alan sitting in front of him, leaning slightly forward, attentive, nodding his head very gently. Dave tried to speak, wanting to say something but softly, still feeling calm and quite unaware how much time had passed. He wanted to say something but it was as if he also didn't want to lose the silence and break the calmness he was feeling. He opened his mouth, and closed it again with a sigh. He blew the breath out of his mouth and took another deep breath. He really didn't know where he had been or what to say.

'Looks like you're struggling for words,' he heard Alan say. He felt himself smile a little. Yes, he thought, I haven't got a clue what to say. He felt a little buzzy. His head felt as though its edges were a bit blurred. He blinked again, slowly this time, another deep breath and slowly sat upright in the chair. 'What was that all about?' he heard himself say. 'I feel as though my head is empty, as if I am sitting in space and I am that space. Does that make any sense?'

Alan could see Dave blinking and he thought Dave looked a little blurred, indistinct somehow. Spatial distortion again. 'Being space?' He knew it didn't make much sense grammatically but that's what he sensed Dave was trying to communicate.

'Whatever that means, but yeah, I don't know what happened, I ... I can't describe it. I was lost in ... in space I guess, but not really lost. I was aware of me somehow but ... but I couldn't sort of think or feel anything. How long was I like that?'

'Nearly ten minutes.'

'I had no sense of time at all, almost like I'd stepped out of time. Where was that place? What was it?'

'Like stepping out of time into another place,' Alan responded, but he didn't add, 'and I am wondering how you are feeling.' He was wondering, but decided to let that ride for now. It would only be directive. Dave seemed more concerned with making sense of what had just happened than exploring how he felt about it, at least for the moment.

'It wasn't scary. It wasn't anything, yet it was so real. I felt a tremendous sense of calm, never felt anything like it before. It felt somehow reassuring, as if, I don't know, a kind of OKness had come over me. Oh, that sounds so silly, but it felt really, really OK to be ... ,' Dave started shaking his head, 'to be wherever I was.'

'Calmness, OKness and reassuring, yes?' Alan could sense something of these qualities in himself. They seemed to be in the room. This was new to him. He thought Dave was going down into a pit and was going to come out with some very different, and probably quite uncomfortable feelings.

'Was it real? Well it must have been. You know, I'm not sure I want to try and analyse it and make sense of it. I just want to let it be. It feels right to just let it be. I don't want to lose the way it has left me feeling. It feels good.' Dave was aware of not wanting these feelings to go, yet he sensed they were beginning to fade away.

'Mhmmm. Just let it be. Maybe we need to just take the rest of the session quietly and allow you to, I don't know, just be with where you are in yourself.' Alan knew that something powerful had happened for Dave, and he knew that sometimes these kinds of experience were, to quote the title of a book he remembered reading many years ago by the mystic Joel Goldsmith, *Beyond Words and Thoughts*. Funny that that had come into his mind. Maybe it's relevant here.

The experienced counsellor learns to trust intuitions. They often come to mind with a sense of 'knowingness' with regard to their relevance. They are often helpful to voice as a kind of offering to the process.

'Beyond words and thoughts,' he said softly.

'Yeah. That really sums it up. Beyond words and thoughts. It is like that. I feel strangely expanded, as if, and this may sound weird, as if I've grown outside of my skin.' Dave couldn't think of any other way of putting it.

'As if you have extended yourself outside of your body?' Alan enquired.

'Yeah, it's a little disorientating. My throat's dry. Any chance of a glass of water?'

'Sure, I'll get you one.' Alan got up and went out to where the water dispenser was. He became aware that his legs felt a little wobbly, and that he was a little spaced out too. He came back with the water, which Dave took and drank slowly. 'That's better. Thanks. Still don't know what else to say.'

'Do you want to say something now, or still want to let it be?' Alan wondered if maybe Dave had shifted a little and wanted to reflect more on the experience.

'I want to let it be. Look, I know we haven't got to the end of the session, but I feel I want to go and spend some time on my own with this. It's not that it isn't helpful being here, but I need time to reflect on my own. Is that OK?' Dave wasn't sure why he wanted this, and it wasn't that he desperately wanted to end the session, but he felt he needed time in his own space to mull over what had happened.

'Sure you're OK?' Alan was feeling concerned at how disorientated Dave may be. 'Or do you want to stay in the room here for a while and I'll pop out and maybe come back when the sessions due to end?' Damn, thought Alan, I'm not trusting him, am I? He added, 'I'm sure you know what feels best for you.'

Dave looked out of the window and thought about it. This room did feel safe, not that he felt unsafe. No, he felt he must move, go for a walk in the park. Felt he needed to get back into his body a bit, as well as reflect on things.

'No, I want to head off, thanks all the same. Same time next week?'

'Actually we had agreed a little earlier so your wife could come along,' Alan replied. Clearly Dave had forgotten.

'Oh yes, OK, 10.00 am, I remember now.' Dave realised he had forgotten that completely.

'Sure you want to stick with that arrangement, Dave, given this experience?'

'Can I phone you and let you know?' Dave felt unsure now about having his wife here. He wanted to think about it and let Alan know.

'Sure, sounds like you may be having second thoughts.' Alan wasn't sure if Dave might have wanted to explore this now.

'Not sure what I'll want. I'll take another drinking diary though. Seems we haven't talked much about drinking this session.'

'That's how it goes sometimes. Did you want to look at anything?' Alan thought it wise to offer the possibility.

'Let me see how I get on. I've made a good start, and that experience just now really has given me some reassuring feelings. I'll try to stick to the current pattern and then we'll look at it next week.' Dave got up. 'Thanks for that,' he said, shaking Alan by the hand. 'It seemed important even though I don't know what it was about!'

'That's OK,' Alan replied, 'and if you need to get in touch, give me a call.'

'Thanks, that's good to know. I feel good. We'll see how the week goes. Bye.'

'Bye, Dave. Take care of yourself.'

Alan watched Dave walk away from the building. Something really deep had happened for Dave. Was it some kind of 'peak experience', the kind that Maslow wrote of? Expanded sense of self, sense of feeling good, calmness, reassurance – it made sense. What a client. Talk about not knowing what was going to happen next. Dave's psychological process seemed to be a bit of a roller-coaster, and he guessed his role was to stay sitting with him when he's on it in the session. He felt a real warmth for Dave. He hoped it was getting across to him in the sessions.

He was aware of being unsure about Dave ending the session early, but he also wanted to respect Dave's choice as well. It was a therapeutic opportunity to convey trust in Dave's own reliance on his own inner prompting. The problem was whether Alan was being congruent. He couldn't play at trusting Dave if he genuinely felt concerned. You couldn't be 'a little bit congruent' when it suited you in therapeutic counselling. Yet Alan saw therapy very much as a process that helped people move towards greater self-reliance and he didn't want to disturb Dave's process of choosing and acting on what he felt to be right for him if he insisted on doing so. The therapeutically helpful response was for the counsellor to congruently express their thoughts and/or feelings whilst acknowledging and supporting the client in whatever choice they make, unconditionally.

Meanwhile, Dave was walking through the park, listening to the birds and thinking how sharp all the colours looked. He found a bench and sat down for a while, taking in the scene around him. The trees seemed so much more alive and the sky, well it seemed a lot more blue somehow. Yes, he felt good. He didn't really know why, he still had to sort out his drinking problem, but he felt good, he felt strong. Alan wasn't so bad, seemed to know what he was about. Felt he could trust him, and that was a good feeling. Felt he cared. Yeah, feeling cared for, that was a big one. And having people to care for as well. He thought of Ian, Emily and Jane. Yeah, people to care for. And of Linda. He smiled and quickened his pace a little. Back to work and then home.

Summary

Dave arrives feeling more positive. He is back with his wife and family. He discusses his drinking diary and his urge to want a drink when out with his son. He mentions how he has talked things through with his wife and she wants to attend the next session. He enters into a place inside himself, which he describes as a pit, and a silence ensues. It proves very powerful and seems to have had a deep effect on Dave, and Alan. Dave leaves feeling much more alive and sensitive to beauty around him, and to his caring feelings for his family.

Points for discussion

- What is the therapeutic value of silence?
- How comfortable do you feel in silence with a client?
- Would you describe Dave's experience as 'spiritual' and how does spirituality connect with counselling theory?
- Powerful sessions can be disorientating for the counsellor. How can focus be regained?
- How can you ensure that intuitive responses are not merely hunches?

Wider focus

- Silences can be awkward, or they can be exactly what a person needs. This is true in any helping relationship. Feeling comfortable in silence is an important quality to develop for when clients need this.
- People also undergo experiences of heightened sensitivity that many would ascribe a 'spiritual' label to. They need to be respected and the client allowed to attach their own meaning to them. They can indicate a turning point, or a liberation from something.

Wednesday morning, 15 November

'Hi Alan, you got my message OK that Linda wasn't coming this week, but plans to come next week?' Dave looked very relaxed, Alan thought, as he came into the counselling room.

'Yes, thanks.'

'I decided I wanted another session on my own to, well, maybe make sense of last week, and to spend time talking strategies which never quite happened last time. I felt I could do this a little easier on my own, although I have talked to her about what happened last week in the session.'

'Fine, so where do you want to start?' Alan asked, keeping it open for Dave to choose his focus.

'I want to look at my drinking. I've done the diaries, and I think I've done well.'

'OK, so what's been happening?' Alan responded as Dave handed him the sheet. 'No lunch-time drinking at all, well done.'

'Yeah, knew I could do it really. I've just got into a different routine, making different choices.'

'And pretty much down to four cans in the evenings, and nothing at all last Wednesday.' Alan wondered how much the experience in the session had contributed to that.

'Yeah, well, after I left here I just felt so good, and I simply didn't feel a need for a drink all evening. Never gave it much thought. Got home, had dinner, talked to Linda about my experience, although I'm not sure what she made of it. I'm still wondering about it myself! Then there was a Morse on TV, one I hadn't seen, and it was soon 10.30 pm and I just didn't feel I needed a drink. Quite an achievement that, given the number of times Morse is either in the bar drinking pints or at home pouring a Scotch! We ended up making love, and that's a first for sometime. Yeah, a really good day.'

Alan was pleased that Dave had handled the TV programme so well. It wasn't easy having something you were trying to give up or cut back on being brought into your living room every night. He had heard many clients with alcohol problems over the years bemoaning the amount of alcohol focus on television. It was a real issue. Imagine trying to give something up, or cut back, whilst it is constantly being brought into your living room.

'So, a dry day, no thoughts of drink, and you made love. As you say, a really good day.' Alan felt really pleased for Dave. And he was aware that Dave, for whatever reason, had not maintained dry the rest of the week. He was sure this would be addressed. For now Dave was feeling good about Wednesday and he, Alan, didn't want to distract him from those feelings. They were, after all, what were present for Dave in the moment, and he wanted to stay with him in those feelings.

'Yeah, so that was Wednesday. Thursday felt good too, decided that I should celebrate. Well, not exactly celebrate, but I felt good, felt I'd cracked it, felt I was OK to have a drink in the evening, felt I was in control. So I had four cans. I didn't rush them, took my time over the course of the evening. And that's pretty much how it has been all week. Getting on well with Linda, and with the kids. It's Ian's birthday this Saturday, he's having a party, ten of his friends coming round. What a nightmare, but I guess it'll be fun too. No, it feels good.'

'So, is that how you feel now, in control, that you've cracked it?'

Alan hoped Dave had but he had seen people crash after a few days, alterations in drinking behaviour having not been sustained because they had not been underpinned by psychological change. Though Dave's experience in the last session had perhaps started the process of change, it was early days. He must keep an open mind, neither optimistic nor pessimistic. Just be there in the therapeutic relationship with Dave.

'Yes, I do. I really feel good about it. Oh, by the way, there's a rush job on at work, I need to head off a little early today if that's OK?'

Alan was experiencing alarm bells going off in his head. Of course, it was up to Dave if he wanted to head off, and if he had work to do then he had to do it. But was he overconfident? Alan decided to see if the alarm bells persisted and, if so, he would say something. If they were fleeting then he'd let them go. He hadn't experienced them this intensely when Dave had left at the previous session. Overconfidence is a definite problem and does put people at risk of lapse or relapse.

'Sure, you need to be where you need to be. When do you need to go?' Alan wanted some clarity on the time boundaries, particularly given the experience of the last session.

'Half past would be great.'

'OK, so 25 minutes left. You wanted to look at strategies first?'

'Yeah. I feel good. I feel in control. I guess I'm wondering whether I need to make any more change. I mean, I feel OK with my drinking now, and it isn't causing problems at home. Linda says she'd rather I drank at home – anyway, stopped her being anxious about what state I might get into in the pub.'

'So she feels things are more under control as well and you are wondering whether you need to make any more changes?' Alan was aware that the alarm bells had not gone away, and that he was feeling a definite unease. He decided not say anything as Dave was focusing on his units and it would cut across it. But he noted it and was prepared to say something later.

'Yeah, I mean, four cans a night isn't much, is it?'

'It doesn't seem so compared to what you were drinking. Of course, it is still above the recommended daily intake.'

'Yeah, I thought you'd say that. Are those figures for real? I mean, four cans, what's that in units?'

'5%, 440 millilitre cans?'

Dave nodded.

'Well that's five times 440 divided by 1000, multiplied by four cans. Uhmmm, that's 8.8 units a day, recommended level is three to four units a day.'

'Think I should reduce further?'

'What do you want to do?'

'I feel OK as I am.' Dave really didn't want to lose his four cans. Hell, he looked forward to them, helped him unwind. He'd achieved a lot. He didn't want to cut back any more.

'You seem very confident, and I really want to acknowledge that, and I have to be honest and say I am concerned as to whether you will sustain this, Dave.'

'Thanks very much. You don't have much faith in me then?'

'Dave, I'm sure you can crack your alcohol problem, I really am, but I have to be honest with you and say that I'm concerned that you could relapse. You know what kind of feelings you have experienced recently, and I guess my concern is whether you would be able to come through those feelings again without a drink.' Alan knew he was taking a risk in one sense, and knew he had to be honest with Dave, who clearly didn't want to hear what he was saying.

'Hmmm,' was all Dave said in response.

Alan thought Dave looked uncomfortable, and somewhat irritated. 'I know it's an uncomfortable thing to have to think about, and it can be somewhat irritating, but I really want to level with you, Dave. I am concerned, and I hope I'm wrong and that my concerns prove to be unfounded,' which pretty much summed up what Alan was feeling.

'OK, but I disagree. Things feel good at home and I feel in control.'

'OK, you disagree and you feel in control.'

Accept what he is saying, Alan said to himself, stay with it. Don't push, he'll only resist. That took him back to his training, hearing a tutor point out that when a client resists it means someone is pushing, and if the only other person in the room is the therapist, then they need to back off and give the client space. People resist for a reason, usually because they are not yet ready to acknowledge something, or feel something. Alan decides to give him some positive reinforcement, this being something he is experiencing as well. He wants Dave to get a sense of the whole of what he is feeling about the situation, not just the concern.

'You're doing well, Dave, you really are, and I'm really pleased that you've got things together at home,' which Alan genuinely felt and so voiced.

'Yeah, I know you mean well, but it really is OK at the moment.' It does feel OK, Dave thought, it really does.

'So, all OK.' Alan was still feeling things were not OK, but couldn't really pin it on to anything in particular.

Dave nodded and added, 'I'll be OK.' A short silence followed before Dave continued, 'And about last week, I still think about that. I still don't know exactly what happened, but I do know it made a profound impact on me. It really did give me a boost.'

'A boost?' Alan hoped Dave would say a little more.

'It sort of gave me a kind of impetus to get things together. Things seemed really clear, somehow. It felt good to be alive.'

Alan suddenly knew what he was feeling so anxious about. It wasn't just the idea of the ending; it was also the party coming up on Saturday, Dave's son's birthday party. What was it Dave had said when he had been talking from his 'lonely me' configuration as David? Hadn't he said that he never had birthday parties? How was Dave going to react on Saturday? Alan was aware that he had drifted off into his own thoughts and Dave had gone silent. Alan realised that he might need to voice these thoughts, particularly if they persisted. In fact, they were getting more intense.

'Good to be alive.' A few moments of silence followed in which Alan became aware that he couldn't let go of his thoughts, so he voiced them. 'Dave, my thoughts just went off to the birthday party Ian's having on Saturday, and I couldn't help remembering something you had said in the session when you really touched into your loneliness, something about you never having birthday parties like all the other children. Was that right?' Alan knew he was directing Dave into a new focus, but he also knew that he needed to say it, that it really was in the way of him hearing Dave, and certainly seemed wholly relevant to what was happening for Dave.

'Yeah, that's right. We're going to make sure Ian has a really good one. No expense spared. And yes, I had thought of that too. I know I didn't have birthday parties, and I'm not going to let my son suffer that too.'

'Sounds really strong. You're not going to let your son suffer like you did.'

'No way. No, I hated missing out as a kid, hated it. Thought there was something wrong with me. Everyone else got things. I didn't. I know what it's like to go without, to feel there's something wrong with you. I'm not going to give that experience to my son.'

'You're damned sure he's not going to miss out like you did.'

'Yeah, I really feel for kids who go without things like that. I know what it's like. They'd ask me when my party was, and I had to make excuses all the time. It was awful. Felt as though I was different to all the others.' Alan noticed Dave was wringing his hands. Dave continued, 'As if I didn't deserve a party, didn't deserve friends. Leaves me feeling cold just thinking about it.'

'Didn't deserve a party or friends, and now left feeling cold.' Alan didn't have to think what to say, the words flowed as a result of the heart connection he felt to Dave as he sat there, clearly disturbed by his memories of a childhood without birthday parties and, it seemed, without many friends. No wonder he was so lonely, not just at home, but probably everywhere. Alan really felt touched by the tragedy of it all.

'Well, my son has lots of friends and he's having a party, and it's going to be a good one.' Alan could see Dave pulling himself away from his own feelings towards his own experience and regaining his focus on Ian and the party to come. He wanted to acknowledge this unvoiced process.

'Hard to focus on your experiences, feels more comfortable thinking about the party on Saturday, I guess.' Again the words flowed from Alan, not so much from thinking about a response, but just a natural reaction to the impression that was affecting him.

'Yeah, two worlds, poles apart. I don't want him to experience what I went through. I want him to have everything I went without.'

'Everything you went without . . . ,' Alan tried not to emphasise the *everything*, as it wasn't the emphasis Dave had given, but this was what Dave picked up on.

It can be so easy to direct a client through tone of voice or intonation. Alan is aware of this and seeks to avoid it, allowing Dave the space to pick up on whatever is most pressing and present for him.

'Yeah, everything. Makes me feel good knowing I'm doing that,' Dave explained, 'makes me feel good.'

'Makes you feel good giving Ian everything you didn't have.' Alan emphasised the *you*.

'But I'm doing it for him really. Just fortunate that it makes me feel good too.' Dave felt he needed to clarify this. Of course he was doing it for Ian, so his son enjoyed himself. It was a bonus that he felt good about it as well, but that was not what he was doing it for. Dave sought to convince himself of this, anyway, although deep down part of himself knew that he was satisfying his own need to feel good. Part of his structure of self needed to gain a sense of satisfaction from knowing he had given his son a good experience. It helped him feel fulfilled, as if his life was to some purpose. Yeah, giving his son lots to smile about made him feel a smile on his face too, and kept those lonely feelings away, although he wasn't actually consciously aware of this part of the process.

Alan picked it up. 'Well, it's making you smile, Dave!'

'Yeah, it's what being a child is all about, having your friends round, playing games, eating too much, you know, jelly and stuff. It'll be great.' Dave could feel his enthusiasm rising as he spoke.

'I hope it goes really well,' Alan replied, so aware that he still had mixed feelings.

Alan could feel Dave's enthusiasm, he seemed to be alive with it. He just hoped all would be well, and that somehow it wouldn't trigger Dave to feel a need to drink to quell his own memories and feelings from childhood should they surface. But he knew he had to trust Dave to know what was best for him. Alan felt that he had been heard when he raised his concerns, even though Dave had brushed them aside. Time would tell. He still had that nagging doubt, though, that this party was going to be a tough experience for Dave, but he could see that Dave was clearly looking forward to it, and wasn't in a place in himself from which he might really hear those doubts.

'Well, time's nearly up. Good luck with the party, and look after yourself. It may be more difficult than you think, but I hope it goes well.'

'Thanks. I do hear your concern, but no, it's going to be great. I'll see you next week with Linda. Is 10.00 am OK?'

'That's fine. I look forward to meeting her and responding to any questions or anxieties she may have, and to hearing about the party as well.'

Alan watched Dave go, and he still had that doubt, but he knew Dave must live his own process, and anyway, maybe he was worrying about nothing. The trouble was, he didn't think so.

Dave felt a spring in his step. It was going to be a good weekend. He knew it. Yeah, he knew that he could feel sad when he thought about his childhood, and he could feel how close it was now, but he could push it away. Saturday was going to be Ian's day, the best he'd ever had. And he, Dave, was going to enjoy it.

It seems likely that Dave is creating and maintaining an unrealistic expectation as a kind of conscious or unconscious reflex to keep himself away from the concerns that Alan has voiced that may be present for him within his sense of self. His own loss of happy birthday experiences is driving his need to fill this emotional and relational void within himself. The question is whether his son's birthday will compensate for what he did not experience. It is unlikely, for it is not his birthday and his friends that are involved. Dave's own sense of loss may come to the surface, which could then lead him to acting in ways that reinforce a belief that he does not deserve treats, or an attempt to compensate by being with his own friends.

Summary

Dave is feeling much more confident after achieving reductions, but Alan is feeling very uneasy when Dave suggests stopping the counselling and talks about his son's birthday party coming up. He voices these concerns and Dave feels angry about it. Alan tries to offer him reassurance that he also sees positive developments, but that he remains concerned. Dave does not want to hear this. The session is shortened as Dave has to return to work. He leaves feeling very positive. Alan is left with his anxiety.

Points for discussion

- Do you agree that a sustainable reduction in alcohol use is likely to require psychological change/personal growth?
- How can a client minimise the impact on them of alcohol use on television or in advertising?
- Was there therapeutic value in Alan voicing his congruent concern towards Dave's intention to stop the counselling?
- The person-centred approach highlights the importance of the counsellor's congruence, unconditional positive regard and empathy for the client's world (which includes both the voiced and unvoiced content). How were these present when Alan expressed his concerns regarding Dave stopping counselling, and the birthday party?
- What do you think is likely to happen to Dave at the party, what choices might he make and what processes will be driving him?

Wider focus

- People can take extreme positions to compensate for, or try to avoid, the psychological discomfort that stems from incongruence.
- All helping professions work with people who can make choices that will put themselves, or what they have achieved, at risk. Concerns can helpfully be voiced in a sensitive but sincere manner. Communicating them alongside awareness of a client's achievements helps to ensure that clients hear the whole perception.

Wednesday morning, 22 November

Linda and Dave arrived together and they sat quietly in the waiting room. Neither spoke to the other. Dave looked anxious. Linda carried an air of simmering anger. Alan came out and noticed that they did not look at ease with each other, and he certainly felt a prickly tension in the air. Oh oh, he thought to himself, something has happened. Well, let's invite them in and see what has been going on.

'Hello, you must be Linda,' he said, putting out his hand which Linda took and shook briefly but firmly.

'Yes, and I'm sure glad to have come this week, although he took some persuading,' she responded, glancing over at Dave with a look of disdain.

'Obviously things have been difficult,' Alan replied, aware they were still in the reception area and really didn't want to get too involved until they were in the counselling room. 'Come on through and sit down, and perhaps we can make some sense of whatever has happened.'

They walked in, Linda ahead, Dave following her, his shoulders tense, staring ahead of him. He didn't look too good, Alan thought to himself.

Alan began by saying to Linda that he hoped to be able to use the session to explain something of the process of resolving alcohol problems, what Dave was working on and why it was difficult to make these kind of changes sometimes. Linda nodded. Dave sat looking at the floor. There was a certain air of haughtiness he felt in Linda's posture. In fact, Alan began to wonder whether she was actually listening to him at all. He ended by saying, 'So, what's been happening and what do you want to use the session for today?'

It was Linda who replied. 'He's useless, can't go a day without a drink. I've had enough. I can't cope. He doesn't help with the kids. He's back down the pub every night. The only reason I haven't thrown him out again is because I thought I'd come here first to tell you what's been happening and get your advice on what to do about him.' The *him* was almost spat out with a kind of venom. Alan didn't want to get into couple counselling – that was not what the session was supposed to be about – but he needed to acknowledge the strength of feeling Linda was expressing.

'So, Dave's been back to the pub and you're ready to throw him out again. I'm wondering what you are hoping for from today?'

'I really don't know. You know what it's like, once an alcoholic always an alcoholic.'

'Is that how you see it, Linda?' Alan knew that he didn't agree with this. It was too simple and did not take into account the uniqueness of each person. Yet he respected it as being Linda's view, and a widely held one as well.

'Yes, I saw it with my father. He was always down the pub, drinking heavily, coming back and then all hell broke loose.'

'You had a tough time as a child with your father's drinking?' Alan empathised with the effect of what Linda had said.

'Yeah, and it's like the pattern repeats itself. Round and round we go. Well, this time I'm not going round any more.' At that Linda put down her bag and took off her coat. It seemed to be a statement of her arrival in the room. She had said her piece and now sat waiting for a response.

'Dave?' Alan asked, looking at where Dave sat, his eyes still down. He hadn't shaved that morning and Alan thought he could smell alcohol. He wanted to invite Dave to speak but not direct him to focus on anything in particular. Obviously, a lot had happened. He wanted Dave to say what he wanted to say. Of course, he was mindful too that Linda's presence might make this difficult for Dave.

'She's right, of course,' Dave spoke quietly. 'I messed up, big time. I've tried to explain to her what happened but she won't listen. Just tells me that "you're all the same".'

'All the same?' Alan was aware he was assuming he meant alcoholics, but he wanted to be sure.

'Alcoholics,' Dave confirmed. 'So it did get out of control . . . .'

'Did get! It *is* out of control,' Linda interjected angrily. Alan was aware that neither was looking at the other during this exchange. Dave lapsed back into silence.

Linda was clearly very angry and emotionally present, Alan noted, but he was mindful of his intention that this should be more of an information exchange than a therapy session. But he could already feel this was not going to be easy. And he also wanted to be open to the process between Dave and Linda and trust that by offering a client-centred relationship growth and understanding could emerge. He wanted to acknowledge Linda but keep the focus on Dave, who was, after all, his client.

'Linda, I really hear your anger, and I also want to hear from Dave what has happened.' He turned to Dave. 'Dave, can you tell me what happened?'

The silence continued and Linda opened her mouth to speak. Alan instinctively lifted his hand and shook his head whilst looking at Linda. She closed her mouth and sat back in the chair.

'You were right. The party got to me. Didn't think it would, but it did. Linda doesn't understand how I was feeling.' Dave looked very sorry for himself as he spoke.

'How were you feeling, Dave?' Alan hoped he might be able to help the communication, which clearly wasn't happening between them.

'The party was great, the kids enjoyed it, and Ian had a great time . . . ,' Dave continued, but was interrupted by Linda.

'Great time. He was in tears during the night . . . .'

'He enjoyed the party. It was what happened after that upset him, I guess.'

'You guess,' Linda replied dismissively, 'I thought it was pretty damn obvious.'

'Yes, OK, I was wrong, for Christ's sake,' Dave's tone of voice sharpened and increased in volume. He was clearly very angry. 'You have done nothing but go on about it. I know it was stupid, it was my fault, but it's done and while I wish it hadn't happened, it has.'

Alan was aware that he hadn't got a clue what they were arguing about, but he could certainly feel the rising irritation in the room. 'Whatever happened has really become a bone of contention, and you're both angry,' he said glancing from Dave to Linda, and back to Dave, wondering who was going to respond.

'I broke his present. We'd got him a new bike, a racer you know with racing wheels and loads of gears and everything.'

'What he isn't telling you is that he came in from the pub, blind drunk, fell over and landed on the bike, buckling the front wheel, scraping the paint and scuffing the seat. A real mess.'

'I didn't do it on purpose, it was an accident,' Dave looked across at Linda, almost pleading with her to hear what he was saying.

'It only happened because you'd been drinking,' Linda retorted, still not looking at Dave.

'So, let me get this clear. Dave went to the pub, came back drunk, fell over and badly damaged the bike. As a result Ian was in tears most of the night.' Alan didn't want to just focus on the events; there were some strong feelings being shown as well. He added, 'And feelings are running high'.

'You know I'm sorry about what happened, I keep saying I'm sorry . . . .'

'Bit late for being sorry, and what have you done ever since – down the pub, every night.'

'Only way to get away from you constantly having a go at me. Can't you let it rest?' Dave had turned to look at Linda who kept her eyes firmly ahead of her.

'So, what's he got to do? Can he go in somewhere, dry out, take some tablets or something?' Linda asked, looking at Alan.

'I hear Linda's anger and I hear you feeling sorry. What do you want, Dave?' Alan asked, not wanting him to feel pushed into anything he didn't want, and concerned that Dave wasn't getting heard in the session by Linda.

'What he wants . . . ,' Linda began. Bloody hell, Alan thought, give him a chance. Alan held up his hand and said, 'I really would like to hear what Dave has to say here.'

I hadn't wanted this to be a kind of therapy session, thought Alan, but this has got to be addressed. I need to give Dave a chance to talk about his thoughts and feelings, and maybe Linda will be able to hear something that she cannot hear when they are reacting to each other at home. Alan could sense Dave's sense of remorse, and he was aware of the temptation to take sides. But Dave was his client; he wanted him to express what he was experiencing.

'I don't know. I feel gutted by it all. I know I shouldn't have gone out to drink after the party, and I didn't mean to damage the bike. But it happened, and I want to understand why. I really don't want it to happen again. I'm as fed up with all this as you are. I hate what's happening, what I'm doing to you, to the kids. I want to get back to some kind of normality, but the truth is, I don't know how to. I just don't know how to.' There were tears in Dave's eyes as he put his head in his hands. 'I really don't know what to do.' The words came out slowly, quietly, and sounded so despairing. Alan looked at him and then across to Linda, who had gone quiet.

'You want to change but you don't know what to do, is that right, Dave?' Alan asked.

'Yeah, I can't go on like this. I really thought I was doing well when I saw you last week. I felt good. I felt in control even though I was still drinking. I felt I was going somewhere with it.'

'You were in control and those feelings were real,' Alan responded, 'and you felt you were going somewhere.'

'And then I blew it. I was so looking forward to Saturday, the party was great, it really went well, didn't it?' Dave looked across at Linda as he finished the sentence.

'Yes, the party was good, Ian did enjoy it and the other children seemed to have a good time,' Linda acknowledged, still staring ahead of her.

Alan wondered whether he should try to get them to look at each other, but decided that this really wasn't what he was there for. They were not in a place in themselves for this, and he must trust their process. He simply wanted to hear what had happened and what they felt about it. He didn't want to embark on couple counselling; that was not the aim of the session. But he did need to help them communicate, and he still didn't really know what had triggered Dave into drinking. He noted to himself how difficult it can be to simply stay with people's feelings and not worry about where it was taking them. But he believed that given a climate of warm acceptance, empathy and genuineness, there was a greater likelihood that somehow the feelings and thoughts that needed to be experienced and expressed would come out. He could see the anger and hurt in both Dave and Linda. Yet they seemed to be acknowledging the positive experience of the party and so he decided to empathise with this.

'So the party went well. All the children were having a good time.' Alan sought to clarify that fact at least.

'Yeah,' Dave responded, 'then I messed up. I don't know what came over me. I'm not sure what happened.' Dave looked up at Alan. 'What was going on, what set me off?' His eyes looked to Alan as if they were searching his own for an answer.

'OK, you messed up, Dave, and I am wondering what had led up to it. Did you sense anything was happening, either of you?'

Alan had sensed that Dave really wanted to understand. The desperate look in his eyes was appealing for answers. Alan was wondering whether Linda may have noticed some changes, or Dave may have felt a build-up of tension or something.

'He started to go quiet around 5.30 pm. I know because I had to start taking more of a lead in organising the kids. Up till then Dave had been organising the games and stuff. I didn't think anything of it at the time, just assumed he was taking a breather.' Linda looked across at Dave, almost looking as though she wanted to know what was happening for Dave. It was the first time she had looked across towards him since the start of the counselling session.

'OK, so your view was that Dave was going quiet, withdrawing, not getting so involved. What was happening for you, Dave?'

Dave sat in silence for a while, trying to figure it out. He didn't know what had happened, but he could remember feeling out of it. He didn't know why, but somehow he had begun to feel uncomfortable. He was feeling it again now. 'It was getting uncomfortable, I'm not sure why. It was after that game, that one where they picked teams and were passing the balloon back and forward along the line.'

'Something about that game, maybe?' Alan enquired. Dave went silent again. Linda opened her mouth as if to say something and Alan shook his head and motioned her to wait.

'I hated team games. It was when Ian's friend, Martin, was picked for that balloon game. He was picked last. There was something I saw in his face, in his expression.' Dave stopped talking and took a deep breath. 'I . . . I was always last to be picked for games at school,' Dave finally said, speaking very slowly and hesitantly. 'No one wanted me in their team. Sometimes they'd argue over who had to have me. It was awful.' Dave lapsed back into silence again.

Linda had never heard Dave speak like this before. She could feel tears in her own eyes as she looked at him, his head bowed, his breaths slow and deep, each out breath released with a sigh that seemed to come from somewhere so deep within him.

'That was a long time ago, Dave,' Linda felt she needed to say something. She could feel her anger beginning to melt away. She had just had no idea that it had been that way for Dave.

'It doesn't feel a long time ago; it feels as real today as it did then somehow. I'd do anything to avoid being left out. I so wanted to be part of things, to feel wanted. But everywhere no one wanted me. I wasn't wanted at home. I wasn't wanted by other kids.'

Linda was reaching out to Dave and putting her arm on his shoulder. Alan felt he needed to acknowledge what Dave had just said, 'You so wanted to feel wanted, but no one. . . .'

'Yeah, always the odd one out, always the one left feeling awkward and forgotten. It hurt so much. Can still feel it.'

'Still hurting, still so in pain.' Alan wanted to let Dave know that he heard the depth of his discomfort, and that it was present now.

Dave took a deep breath and let out a sigh. 'Yeah, but it's no excuse for what happened.'

'What happened?' Alan tried to make it sound like a reflection but he knew it was really a question.

'As soon as all the children had gone I went down to the pub. I just went. I didn't give it any thought. I didn't try and stop myself or think rationally. I just went. I knew I just had to go and get a drink.'

'Just knew I had to get a drink.' A thought crossed Alan's mind, which left him puzzled. The more he tried to push the thought away, the more solid it seemed to become. He voiced it. 'Why the pub?'

'Friends there,' Dave replied without hesitation. He looked up, surprised by what he had said. 'Friends there,' he said again.

'Friends there?' Alan was aware that he had become very focused on Dave and felt himself wondering what Linda might be feeling, or how she might be looking. But he wanted to maintain his connection with Dave.

'Yeah, it just felt important to be with them. I knew they'd be there and I knew they'd be pleased to see me.'

The last eight words stuck with Alan, he sensed their importance and reflected them back, 'I knew they'd be pleased to see me.'

Alan preferred to reflect in the first person. It always seemed a much more powerful affirmation of what the client was trying to say, to express, from within his or her inner world. He would often reflect back slowly and, where appropriate, quietly so as not to disturb the client's focus.

'I needed to be with friends, with . . . .' Dave stopped speaking. He didn't know what to say. He could feel himself stopping and silence creeping over him. He was aware of his own stillness, of sitting not able to move, not wanting to move. He sat. He could feel his heart pounding and churning sensations just beneath his chest. Tears welled up in his eyes, hot, burning tears. He couldn't stop them. Waves of emotion swept through and over him, a deep longing and a wanting for friends. He dropped his head. The tears kept flowing. He could hear sounds coming from his throat. His breath was in short bursts. He tried to swallow back the tears, the feelings that were surging through him, but he could not. He felt powerless. He felt a hand rubbing his arm, it seemed so far away, he reached across for it with his other hand, the tears just kept flowing out, as if some great vat of water had been breached somewhere deep inside himself. He gripped the hand on his arm.

Linda had never witnessed anything like this, and certainly not from Dave. She felt so many different feelings and emotions. Sadness for the pain she sensed Dave must be going through; fear for what was going to happen next; love for the man who, whilst he irritated her and gave her such a hard time, she realised she still cared deeply for. Oh Dave, she thought, you stupid, wonderful idiot.

Alan sat holding himself open to the thoughts and feelings impressing on his awareness whilst consciously allowing his heart to go out to Dave in his place of despair and desolation. There were no surging energies in Alan, but there was a steady and gentle compassion, a caring for Dave as he sat amidst the storm. Words of wisdom he had read many years before came into his mind, 'Look for the flower to bloom in the silence that follows the storm: not till then.' He just noticed their presence in his mind. They were not pressing, he did not feel a need to voice them, but they somehow left him with a kind of reassurance that all was somehow OK. Sometimes thoughts may not carry an urge to be voiced, and this should be respected.

The tears began to subside and Dave found a strange calm descending on him once again. He blinked and took a few deep breaths, slowly lifted his head and looked to Linda. She was looking back at him with tears in her eyes. He tried to smile but the lump returned to his throat again. He turned towards Alan. 'Friends, I needed friends. I saw Ian with his friends and remember feeling so pleased for him, but there was something in me that was empty. The more I saw Ian playing with his friends, the more empty I realised I was.'

'So empty,' Alan responded, keeping it short, empathically sensing Dave's need not to have his flow interrupted.

Brief, empathic responses are often the most powerful, but can be difficult. Saying something briefly can affirm that the client has been heard but without interrupting the flow.

'Yeah. Gradually it began to overwhelm me. That was when I went quiet at the party and started to withdraw. I was full of emptiness. And then seeing the expression on Martin's face when they were picking teams.'

Alan responded with, 'That expression on Martin's face. So full of emptiness,' and then heard himself add, 'your emptiness was overflowing,' which he hadn't planned to say.

'Overflowing with emptiness, yeah, that just about sums it up. Jeez I like that, *overflowing with emptiness*. I had to get away from it. I had to go and find my friends.'

'Oh darling,' Linda was saying, 'I didn't understand. If only you had said something, maybe I might have . . . ,' but Dave interrupted.

'I wouldn't have heard you. I couldn't hear anything but what was happening inside me. That's what's so scary. I had no control, Alan, I had no control. How can I get control? I don't want this to happen again.' Dave looked at Alan who looked back and reflected Dave's fear.

'No control, mustn't let it happen again.'

'I need help, Alan. I know it's down to me, but I need help. I hurt inside so much and I've got to resolve it. But it will be so hard to do it and not drink. But I have to. I really have to.'

'I hear you Dave. I hear the desperation. You want to resolve that hurt. You want to stop hurting.'

'It feels so scary. I'm going to need your help too, Linda. I need you to understand.'

'I want to try to understand, but it is hard. I don't feel a need for a drink when I'm hurting inside, I don't understand why you do, why you can't stop yourself.' Linda was looking intently at Dave now as she spoke to him. Her words were very gentle and warm.

'It's hard to understand from the outside,' Alan commented to Linda. 'It can seem to not make any sense, but in the moment for Dave, getting that drink seems the most logical thing in the world. Yet I am also aware that this time it wasn't the drink that was uppermost in your mind, it was being with friends.'

Alan was wondering whether this was helpful or not, but whilst Dave had ended up drinking he had been saying for the last few minutes he was going out looking for his friends rather than looking for a drink. It seemed important to clarify this, particularly as it is so difficult to understand when a decision leads to a drinking episode. Sometimes it is made with the intention to drink, sometimes not.

'The drink happened 'cos I was in the pub. I went out to be with people. But then it all got crazy.'

'Do you think you were planning to drink heavily?' Alan asked.

'I don't know. Funny, but I kind of knew I would but somehow wasn't planning to. Doesn't make sense.'

'As though part of you simply wanted to be with friends to ease the emptiness, but another part of you was almost waiting to take advantage of the situation and trigger you into heavy drinking?' Alan asked, trying desperately to clarify his sense of what may have been going on for Dave.

'Sounds weird, but the empty bit of me was looking for friends. I'm not sure it was looking for a drink.'

Alan was curious. 'So friends fill the emptiness rather than alcohol?'

'Ye-es,' Dave was also intrigued now. Did he drink on emptiness? What was it they had recognised in that earlier session, that he drank on his sense of *lonely me*. Lonely me, empty me, how many me's are there, he wondered! A sudden insight rushed in on him. He voiced it. 'I drink on lonely me, but loneliness feels so close to emptiness, they run into each other. I can't tell them apart. I guess I was lonely at that party, yeah, it's like feeling lonely makes me feel empty, but feeling empty make me feel lonely. Yeah. And alcohol helps me to dull it all.'

'Loneliness leads to emptiness. Emptiness leads to loneliness. Alcohol dulls them both,' Alan replied, feeling good that Dave was making his own connections.

The client is going to find it much more therapeutically powerful to be allowed the space to do this than the therapist making connections for them. The insight can be owned. It is the client's truth, and it can encourage the client to engage further in self-reflection.

'Yeah, alcohol makes me feel good.'

'It's the alcohol that makes you feel good,' Alan responded, aware that he had sensed a thought passing through his mind as to whether it was the alcohol doing this alone, or whether it needed to be in combination with other people being around to interact with, like Dave's friends down the pub, or Linda at home when they were on good terms.

Dave was quiet again. It was Linda who spoke. 'I never realised you were so lonely, Dave. I can't say I understand it, and I don't know what to do about it. Why alcohol, though?'

'It made me feel good. When I was out with friends, I felt part of something, felt confident, felt a buzz. But I never drank with the intention of avoiding feeling lonely.'

'Never?' Alan replied, the word leaving all three of them in a moment of silence before Dave responded, aware that he was feeling uncomfortable again.

'Hmmm. I guess I need to think about that. I suppose I mean, I went to the pub with my mates to have a few laughs, you know, like you do.'

'Seemed more like to get away from me and the kids,' Linda cut in.

'I'm talking about the past, before we met, not now. It's different now. You moan about me going down the pub, just makes me want to go down even more.' Dave could feel irritation rising in himself. Here we go, he thought.

'What else can I do? You leave me with the kids, come back pissed whenever you feel like it. Spend money we can't afford. How do you expect me to react? How do you think I feel when you go out?' Linda was looking not so much angry as distraught. Alan wondered why, and wondered whether to respond. It was Dave's session but things were happening here between them and he felt he wanted to respond.

'Dave, I hear the irritation in your voice, and I hear your distress, Linda, at the thought of Dave going down to the pub. I wonder if it is this kind of exchange that typifies how it can be for you both at home.' Alan hoped he had managed to touch both Dave's and Linda's inner worlds. He wondered who would reply first.

Alan was aware that he did not know who to focus on, so he trusted that the process of communication taking place would lead to whatever needed to be said being voiced, whether Linda or Dave. Alan is now definitely giving Linda space to disclose something. Linda looking distraught has made an impression on him. The therapeutic focus may now shift to her. Alan has made this possible in response to his experience of being in relationship with Dave and Linda.

It might be argued that he has encouraged disclosure from Linda with whom he does not have a counselling contract. Sometimes, in the moment, and within the relational experience, the unfolding process has to be trusted. Alan therefore continues to offer empathy, warm acceptance and to maintain his congruence. He seeks to continue to foster a climate of safety through his words, attentiveness, body posture and facial expression.

It was Linda. 'I had to put up with my father going down the pub every night, getting drunk, coming home, being abusive to my mother. He hit her a lot. It was awful.' She dropped her voice and said quietly, 'Sometimes I got it as well.' She paused, and continued, 'night after night.' There were tears in Linda's eyes. 'I can't cope with you coming home drunk, Dave. I can't cope with it. I know you're hurting inside, and so am I.'

Dave looked surprised. 'You never said, I mean, I knew you'd had a tough time at home, but . . . you never said.'

'You'd never told Dave this, Linda? And you've never heard this, Dave?' Alan waited again to see who would respond. He wanted to respect the interaction between Linda and Dave and allow it to continue. They had stuff they needed to talk about.

'I didn't know. I really didn't know he'd knocked you and your mother about. The bastard.' Dave went quiet for a moment and then added, 'But I'm not your father.'

'Doesn't stop me feeling scared when you go out,' Linda replied in a quiet voice, tears beginning to slide down her cheeks.

They both lapsed into silence. Neither knew what to say. It was Dave who made the first move, reaching over and taking her hand. He felt awkward, he knew he was being tentative, and he knew that he wanted to be more forthcoming, but he had always found it difficult to show feelings.

Alan's empathic response was to honour the silence. He recognised Dave's hesitancy in reaching out. He felt they needed to be in touch with each other in this moment. He noticed Linda squeezing his hand, tears were still running down her face. Alan wondered when was the last time they had shared such a tender moment. He didn't know, and didn't want to make assumptions. He allowed them to be together.

The therapist can communicate silence to the client as a way of empathising with the silence that they are communicating. A lot can be said non-verbally in a silence. This was a silence shared between Dave and Linda and it was not for him, Alan, to get in the way of it.

'I'm sorry,' Linda finally said, dabbing her cheeks and her eyes with a tissue.

Dave smiled at her. 'No need to feel sorry, love, but I guess it isn't easy to be with the feelings that are with you,' as he noted Linda's unease.

'It seems we are both a bit sensitive today,' she half-smiled, and turned to look at Dave, who was looking at her and still holding her hand.

'A lot of sensitivity which you have shared with each other,' Alan said quietly.

This was the aspect that had impressed itself on Alan, and he wanted to acknowledge it. It seemed as though the honesty Linda and Dave had shown each other about their feelings had drawn them closer together. He felt privileged to have been part of their process, but he knew as well that there was a long way to go. Both were carrying strong sensitivities linked to their pasts. Each had been faced with childhood experiences that had left emotional scars. Hearing what Linda had said about her fear as she waited for her drunken father to return was a story he had heard many times. He knew that adults who as children had experienced the uncertainty and the unpredictability that stemmed from being in a chaotic and disharmonious family environment were left with a higher risk of problems later in adult life (Velleman and Orford, 1993). As an adult there was a high risk of them seeking a relationship that would perpetuate what had been internalised as a child as 'normal' experience. Linda had chosen to be with Dave, a person struggling to be emotionally available as he had spent a childhood himself bereft of emotional contact. Seeing them together, tentatively allowing very caring human feelings to be present between them was heart-warming. A first step, perhaps, towards each of them taking the steps needed to resolve their underlying sensitivities and to rebuild themselves to become more resilient to the feelings that currently could so easily overwhelm them.

'This feels like an important first step.' Alan wanted to acknowledge and make present his sense that they were embarking on a long road to recovering from the damage that each had suffered. He wanted to be transparent to them, to allow his sense of the importance of what had occurred to be clearly visible as he sat in therapeutic relationship with Dave and Linda.

They were both nodding.

'It won't be easy,' Dave acknowledged, 'and I am still not too sure what to do about my drinking. But I do know I want to change. And I want to work at it with you,' looking at Linda, 'and you,' looking at Alan.

Alan nodded. He didn't feel he needed to say anything. There was a common knowing in the room. 'You really want to turn things around, Dave. And I hear you saying you're not sure what to do about your drinking.' Alan was wondering whether to focus on some strategies for the coming week, or to acknowledge Dave's not knowing what to do, when Linda spoke.

'I think I need to look at myself as well, and try to make sense of my past and how it is affecting me now. What do you think?' she looked at Alan.

'That is what you feel you want to do?' Alan asked, wanting to hold Linda with her decision and to be sure he really was in touch with what she wanted.

'Yes, Dave may be the one drinking, but I'm contributing. And it does affect me so I need to think about all this, and I need some ideas about what to do and how to be with Dave to help him. How can I not react? What if he wants to go down the pub again and I can't control my feelings?'

Alan noticed the fear in Linda's eyes, or at least what he took to be fear. He wanted to be clear. 'You look quite fearful about your reactions and not being able to control your feelings.'

'I want to help Dave, but I need some ideas.'

'How do you feel about that Dave? We could spend a few minutes on this, or is there something else you want to focus on?' Alan was aware that it was an opportunity as Linda was here to 'brainstorm' ways of responding to Dave should he show signs of acting on an urge to go out drinking.

'Yeah, and maybe some ideas to help me will come out of it too,' Dave replied.

'So, where shall we start?' Alan was not sure what aspect Linda or Dave would want to focus on.

'I guess I'm concerned about situations that can leave me wanting to go down the pub. I need to learn to handle feelings better. I know feeling lonely is a major trigger. I can't stop feeling lonely sometimes, but I have to learn to react differently.'

Alan nodded. 'Seems like you need to somehow give yourself time to choose a response to those feelings rather than follow an instinctive reaction,' Alan responded.

Dave nodded and sat reflecting for a few moments.

Alan recognised that this was not really empathic to how Dave had described it. Yet he was also aware of the situation, that Dave had wanted to focus on ideas to help him to handle his feelings and minimise the risk of further drinking episodes. His comment had come into his mind almost instinctively; it was a perception that often had relevance with clients with alcohol problems like this. So he recognised it had come from his own experience, but that it had been drawn out by Dave's comment. It had felt appropriate as he sat there listening to Dave and being open to his own feelings and thoughts.

Alan found himself struck with a kind of wondering about what went on between Linda and Dave before he went to the pub. Was there a build up of tension in the relationship, or was it simply Dave's internal clock telling him it was time for a drink, or maybe something else. Before he had an opportunity to voice this, Dave spoke.

'I need to be able to think, not react,' was his response.

'It never feels as if you are thinking anything other than going for that drink and being with your friends down at the pub,' asked Linda as she looked across to Dave, who was nodding.

'Part of it is habit. I think often it is habit. I don't experience the strong feelings of loneliness every time,' Dave replied.

'Maybe the habit reaction cuts in before you have a chance to really experience the depth of loneliness that may be present?' Alan asked, being aware that habitual drinking by the clock can mask underlying needs. He wasn't sure if this was how it was for Dave. He wanted to get clear in his own mind how Dave was experiencing it.

'It usually feels pretty tense. Well I feel tense after we have eaten each night, wondering what will happen,' Linda added before Dave had a chance to reply.

'So you are feeling tense Linda and then . . . ?' Alan left the question hanging.

'Dave usually has some reason why he needs to see someone.'

'Well, sometimes I do, and sometimes it is just an excuse. But you often say that you suppose I'm going to get pissed again tonight, and that makes me feel angry.'

'Angry.' Alan could sense its presence as Dave spoke.

'Yeah, angry. It really hurts. It feels like . . . .' Dave's voice trailed off as he thought for a moment.

'Feels like?' Alan responded wanting to give Dave time to explore this feeling.

'Makes me uncomfortable. Yeah, OK, sometimes I make an excuse, but it's the way you say it. A real put-down, as if I'm doing something wrong.'

'So you hear it as a put-down as if you have done something wrong?' Alan reflected, but with a questioning intonation as he spoke.

'Yeah, makes me feel even more like I want to go down the pub.'

'OK.' Alan realised he was not sure of something and he wanted to be clear. 'So what Linda says makes you feel more like going down the pub. Do you mean more like getting out the house and the pub is where you go, or more like having a drink, or maybe both?'

Dave thought about it for a moment. 'More like going and getting a drink.'

'And you are choosing to go out for that drink rather than have it at home?' Alan asked.

'Yeah, except for when I tried cutting back recently, but then it seemed easier somehow.'

'It seemed easier?' Again Alan reflected as a question.

'Things felt more comfortable between us. I didn't feel the need to go out. I felt OK being at home with my cans.'

Alan was wondering what had changed then to allow this to happen. What was meant by feeling more comfortable? 'So feeling more comfortable reduced the need to go out?'

'Yeah. I mean, it wasn't easy, but I wanted to stay in. I knew it wasn't doing me any good going out drinking every night and drinking at home helped me drink less. I missed being with people, but not enough to make me go out. There were some things on TV that helped as well I remember, a couple of good films and some football. Kept me focused.'

'So things to focus on helped,' Alan replied.

'Yeah, and I need to get back to that.'

'You could read the children a story, Dave. They miss you when you're not there in the evenings,' Linda responded. 'We could do some stuff together as well. It would be good for us.'

'How does that seem for you, Dave?' Alan asked.

Dave was nodding. 'I could do that, and maybe we do need to do things together in the evenings. We used to but I guess we got out of the habit.'

'OK, so work at doing things together and Dave to spend time with the children. And maybe you'll come up with some other ideas.'

Alan had noticed that the time was nearly up, and he did not feel it therefore appropriate to start empathising with how they had got out of the habit of doing things together. So he put in the brief summary and then drew attention to the time.

'We only have a couple of minutes left. Anything else?'

'What if Dave insists on going to the pub? What can I do then?' Linda asked.

'I won't,' Dave reacted.

'Dave, I want to be realistic. What if something happens and you do decide to go, what then?' she persisted.

Dave said nothing but he looked awkward. 'Dave, what would make you stop and think?' Alan asked.

'I don't know, I suppose I'd need to be reminded of what we have decided here, but it wouldn't be any good trying to pressure me.' Dave knew when he was in that frame of mind he couldn't be told what to do, that he was more likely to react and do what he was being pressured into not doing.

Alan had offered a technique to couples before with this kind of problem and he felt it appropriate to offer it here. 'Sometimes agreeing a word or a phrase which when either of you says it means one of you is concerned and needs to call a halt to whatever is happening or being said. Something unusual, maybe something that might make you both smile.' Alan suddenly remembered one couple that had hit on the idea of using his name! If either was feeling a need to stop an exchange of words they would shout 'Alan!' The crazy thing was that it had actually helped them.

'Aardvark, that's a word that's always seemed funny to me,' Dave suggested.

'Where did that come from?' Linda replied, looking somewhat taken aback, but smiling.

'Don't know. Remember hearing a joke once, and aardvark was in the punch line. Can't remember it now though.'

'OK,' replied Linda, 'aardvark it is. What the hell is an aardvark anyway?'

'Some kind of animal, I think,' Dave replied. He looked at Alan.

'Don't ask me, you're probably right. Sounds like the first thing you're doing together tonight is getting out the dictionary!' Alan couldn't resist that quip. Well, it triggered smiles around the room.

The session came to an end and Dave agreed to come back the following week at 11.00 am and again to try and complete a drinking diary for the week. Linda felt she didn't need to come back but wanted the option of coming with Dave another time if they both felt it would be helpful at the time. Alan agreed to that.

They left and Alan noticed them walking across the car park and talking. Well, it has been stormy for them both but maybe they have a chance now to put some of that behind them, he thought as he watched from the window.

Now, what was that passage that had come to mind earlier? Oh yes, 'Look for the flower to bloom in the silence that follows the storm: not till then.' He went to find the book that he had remembered it from. He felt he needed to reconnect with the whole passage. Yes, there it was, he read it to himself, allowing the words to enter deep into his being:

"Look for the flower to bloom in the silence that follows the storm: not till then. It shall grow, it will shoot up, it will make branches and leaves and form buds, while the storm continues, while the battle lasts. But not till the whole personality of the man is dissolved and melted – not until it is held by the divine fragment which has created it, as a mere subject for grave experiment and experience – not until the whole nature has yielded and can become subject unto its Higher Self, can the bloom open. Then will come a calm such as comes in a tropical country after the heavy rain, when Nature works so swiftly that one may see her action. Such a calm will come to the harassed spirit. And in the deep silence the mysterious event will occur which will prove that the way has been found. Call it by what you will, it is a voice that speaks where there is none to speak – it is a messenger that comes, a messenger without form or substance; or it is the flower of the soul that is opened. It cannot be described by any metaphor. But it can be felt after, looked

for, and desired, even amid the raging of the storm. The silence may last a moment of time or it may last a thousand years. But it will end. Yet you will carry its strength with you. Again and again the battle must be fought and won. It is only for an interval that Nature can be still.'' (MC, 1920, pp. 13–15)

Alan slowly put the book down, there were tears in his eyes and a gentle knowing lodged deep in his heart. Yes, I needed to read that again, for myself. 'Again and again the battle must be fought and won', that sounded like the struggle to overcome addiction. How many times would Dave have to battle to finally get control he wondered? Lapses and relapses are part of the 'Cycle of Change' (Prochaska and DiClemente, 1982) and he hoped Dave would not need to encounter too many.

Summary

What had been planned by Alan as an information session did become couple counselling. Dave had drunk heavily following his son's party and had broken his son's new bicycle. Linda is angry. Dave discloses his loneliness and his struggle to have friends as a child. Linda is deeply moved and discloses her father's drunken behaviour when she was a child. It brings them closer together. They come out of it feeling more united and wanting to work together to help Dave overcome his alcohol use.

Points for discussion

- Was it appropriate that the session evolved into couple counselling and, if so, why?
- On a number of occasions, Alan indicated to Linda not to say anything. He also experienced irritation with her. Was this appropriate?
- How do you think you would have felt being the counsellor in this session? Would you have felt able to maintain impartiality?
- What were the key responses or facilitative actions by Alan, if any, that enabled Dave and Linda to come closer together when they arrived so far apart?

Wider issues

Working with couples is often helpful in this kind of scenario, though not always possible as the client's partner may not want to be involved, sometimes seeing it as 'not my problem'. Often, however, there are issues of co-dependency. Professionals not confident in working with couples may need to refer on. Generally, much help can be offered by simply enabling couples to communicate with each other. What is vital is not to take sides.

Friday afternoon, 24 November

'Good job we talked about couple counselling last time,' Alan said as he settled
into the easy chair in Jan's counselling room. 'Not that it turned out how we
discussed, and it did end up as couple counselling at times and not just information exchange, but it was very powerful and deeply moving. Made a big impression on me and left me feeling quite drained. I was glad to have given myself
extra time after that session before the next person. I had half an hour and I
really needed it.'
'So, what happened?' Jan enquired.
'Dave came with his wife, Linda, but I am also aware that there were some other
things that have happened in previous sessions that I want to talk about, so I'm
not sure where to begin.'

Alan was thinking back to the sessions when Dave had experienced that
dark pit and yet curiously ended up with a strong sense of calm and of feeling
OK. He wanted to check that assumption he had made about Dave being
in the pit. And there was everything about the birthday party, Dave's confidence and his, Alan's, feeling that it was going to be a problem, as well
as that session with Linda. The last session was fresh in his mind, but there
was something about that calmness Dave had touched that was very
present in his thoughts.

Jan sensed that Alan was not sure where to start. She didn't want to direct him,
but she wanted to acknowledge her sense. 'Seems like there is a lot of material
and I guess it has made a strong impact on you. Hard to know where to start?'
she asked, leaving Alan to pick up the story where he felt he needed to.
'So much seems to be going on for Dave at the moment. He really does seem to be
moving across a whole range of experiences. It is almost as though he is connecting with parts of himself, and my sense is that there is some kind of process
running here.'
'Some kind of process that is helping Dave feel more connected with himself?' Jan
asked, wanting to be sure she was clear on what Alan was saying, and allowing
Alan to hear it himself so he could clarify anything that did not sound right.

'The session after the last supervision, Dave went into himself and into what he described as being a deep, dark pit. I immediately thought he was descending into some dark depth, and I remember responding: "A deep, dark pit. You inside it?" But he corrected me saying, "No, it's inside me." I had assumed it was his whole self entering into a pit.'

'Any idea where that assumption came from? Can you remember whether you felt connected with Dave at the time?' Jan was wondering whether Alan was speaking from his own experience.

'I thought I was,' Alan replied, trying to remember how he had felt.

Alan had spent time reflecting on this himself. He regularly used a period of self-reflection to process his counselling work. He found this an important discipline and aid to helping him understand his own process and what was happening in the sessions rather than simply always waiting for the next supervision session. He felt it was a responsibility of counsellors to self-monitor. However, in this case he had struggled to get clarity as to his feelings and sense of what had been happening in the session with Dave.

'What was being talked about before you made your assumption?'

'We were talking about how empty he would feel if he had to face not being with his wife and children. It was emptiness that took him into the pit.'

'You are doing it again,' Jan replied, 'talking of him going into the pit, even though you say he said the pit was in him.'

'Dammit, something's going on here and I need to clear it.'

'Emptiness,' Jan said it softly, 'where does emptiness take you?'

Alan sat and thought, but not for long. He knew it was his own relationship break-up that had dropped him into the pit. 'It's my stuff. It was my experience, but somehow at the time and after I didn't think of it, it just seemed so reasonable to assume Dave as a whole was dropping into a pit,' he said finally, feeling irritated that his own stuff was clouding his sensitivity to his client. Alan had not experienced this himself for some time. He had done a lot of work on himself in order to move on, yet it seemed that scars remained. 'It seems that even though I have come to terms with what happened, it was so intense that I have a kind of weak spot, and themes that come up, or feelings that become present that touch into that part of me, trigger this kind of assumption.' Alan was annoyed with himself.

'You don't look very comfortable,' Jan replied, knowing that Alan set high standards for himself and that he didn't like to feel he was not clear in himself in his therapeutic work.

'I've been working on my sense of loneliness in therapy, and it has been really helpful. I am annoyed that something like this got past me. I'm going to look at this more, but not here. I am wondering, though, what reaction you have to this?'

'I'm sitting with a sense of just how close some of Dave's experiencing is to yours, and how you need to be aware of this in working with him. It seems as though

Dave corrected you pretty quickly and no harm was done. He explained how it was and presumably you moved on into his world of experience. I am assuming – it seems assumptions are in the air today – that your assumption didn't stick with you.'

Jan noted how, in supervision, the supervisor could parallel in some way the issues within the counselling sessions. Her job was to try and notice these and highlight them. They often had meaning. Assumption seemed to be emerging as a theme and she wondered what relevance it might have both to Alan's relationship to Dave, and to Dave generally in his life. It sometimes felt like she was taking a position just behind the counsellor, ready to catch anything emanating from the client that the counsellor missed, yet holding a vantage point so that she might sense what impact the counsellor might be having on the client. Yet she knew, too, how reliant she was on the counsellor being open. Therefore she sought to create a collaborative environment so that she and Alan could work together as co-professionals, not in some kind of teacher–pupil relationship.

'It didn't stick. As I recall, Dave moved on and connected with the pit inside himself.'

'So how do you think the theme of *assumptions* may have relevance in your relationship to Dave, or in Dave's life in general?'

'I'm not sure. I was aware pretty quickly that I was making an assumption when it happened. I suppose when Dave spoke of his assumption that he would be OK at his son's birthday party.'

Jan looked curious, 'What happened with his son's birthday party?' she asked.

'Well this was the next session. His son was having a birthday party on the Saturday and Dave was looking forward to it, to giving his son the kind of birthday he didn't have as a child. I felt alarm bells and tried to voice my concern, but he would have none of it. He was sure he would be OK. He assumed he was going to be able to cope.'

'And did he?' Jan knew the answer before she asked the question.

'Well, he used alcohol to cope – let's put it that way – and the last session with Linda was following the birthday party. Dave had been affected and had felt an urge to be with his friends seeing his son having fun with *his* friends and in particular when sides were being picked for a team game it took him back to his own painful memories of not being picked till last. Dave ended up in the pub, drinking heavily, and it triggered a relapse for a few days back to pub drinking. Before then he had got it back under some degree of control and was working at cutting back further.'

'So, Dave made an assumption about his ability to control his drinking in what must have been a difficult situation at some level for him. Maybe he makes assumptions about a lot of things? It may be something to be aware of, and which may need to be highlighted if it feels to be a factor when you are with him again.'

Jan didn't want to suggest Alan raised it as, like Alan, she did not believe in being directive and going into sessions with a pre-planned list of items that had to be covered. So often clients have moved to a different place, and the person-centred approach honours this. She believed things should be raised when they were felt to be part of the therapeutic process. She strongly liked the concept of *transparency* as a description of congruence and the ability of the therapist to voice experiences that became present within them during, and as a product of, the therapeutic relationship.

'Yes, I think I need to carry a heightened awareness of it, and see what happens. The problem in this line of work, particularly with alcohol problems, is that people can easily make lots of assumptions. You only have to say the word "alcoholic" and a whole host of images can come to a person's mind that may have no relevance whatsoever to the person who is being referred to. And, of course, Dave's childhood was riddled with assumptions as he tried to make sense of his relationship with his mother. He clearly assumed that loneliness and rejection were somehow normal, or at least, normal for him to experience. The more I think about this now, the more this theme of assumptions makes sense. But not just for Dave. It is a factor for so many clients, well, for all of us, isn't it? We start making assumptions at such an early age as we try to make sense of our experiences.'

Alan was thinking of a number of his clients who had all made natural assumptions in childhood because of what they experienced of never being good enough or of not deserving to feel happy. This could be the result of many experiences, and themes that often emerge are: violence in the home, victimisation, physical and sexual abuse, lack of prizing or constant criticism. As children we receive a lot of negative experiencing that we try to make sense of, and often the sense that is made involves the belief that we deserve to feel hurt because of who we are, and this then becomes a 'configuration of self' within the individual's self-concept. This then fuels assumptions that we make about ourselves in later life, often resulting in a reinforcement of the original attempt to make sense of a dysfunctional situation.

It is always somebody else's 'good enough' that we are supposed to conform to, Alan thought, producing what Rogers termed *conditions of worth*. 'I'm thinking of conditions of worth,' Alan added, 'and acknowledging their link with making assumptions.'

'How do you see, or maybe I should say experience, Dave's conditions of worth?' Jan asked.

'Nice one!' was Alan's instant response. So, what had Dave been conditioned into in order to feel some degree of worth? 'Well, he said he got no cuddles from his mother, no parties, no friends to speak of. He has also told me how he never got picked for teams at school, that he was always the last to be picked and really neither side wanted him. It must have seemed such an impossible idea for Dave to feel accepted, wanted and cared for. The more I think of it now, the more angry I feel about what he had to go through. I often think that if I had had the experiences of my clients maybe I would be drinking heavily to cope, and I certainly think that with Dave. With his background, I might have handled my relationship break-up last year in a very different way. Makes you think. Makes me feel quite humble, somehow.'

'Humble?'

'Maybe that's the wrong word, I don't know, but it makes me aware of just how fortunate I am and not because of anything that I kind of achieved. I didn't have Dave's early experiences and so I wasn't left with the sensitivities that he has, or at least not the associated habit reactions that he has with them of taking alcohol to quell uncomfortable feelings. Me, I just headed off to the gym and burned it off when I was struggling last year. But it could have been very different. Makes you think.' Alan sat for a moment, aware of how awesome this kind of thinking was.

'Makes *you* think,' he heard Jan say. Yes it did make him think, it made him very aware that if life experiences had been reversed it could have been Dave counselling him for a drink problem!

'One of the things I always try to get across in training is this idea that there is no *us and them* with problem drinking. We are all human beings trying to make the best of things, and some of us choose alcohol to help, because it eases the pain, or gives us a boost, or a good feeling.'

Jan knew from past conversations that Alan felt this way, and she could sense his feeling for Dave. It was very present and she voiced it. 'You really feel for Dave, don't you?'

'I do, and it was very present for me when he was with Linda early on in the session. He had relapsed and she was giving him a hard time in the session. At the time I didn't appreciate the background and sensitivities. What I felt was that I wanted her to shut up and give Dave some space.'

'Sounds as though you were maybe being a bit protective of Dave against Linda?' Jan suggested.

That hadn't occurred to Alan. A broad grin broke out on his face. 'Never thought of myself as a mother hen before,' he replied and broke out laughing. 'But the session changed later and they really came together. It was very moving. Dave talked about his loneliness and the rejections he had had in childhood, particularly the experiences around not having friends, not being popular, and Linda talked of her father who had an alcohol problem and the arguments at home when he came back from the pub. They both heard things they hadn't heard before, and it really drew them together.'

'Sounds like a good piece of work.'

'Didn't feel like work. I didn't really say much, or at least I don't remember it as though I did. I remember wanting to let them be in the moment, particularly when Dave reached out to take Linda's hand when she had been talking about how much fear she had linking back to her father going down the pub and coming back drunk, and how this connected to Dave going down the pub.' Alan sensed water in his own eyes as he related this part of the session. It had been so touching, and he felt as if he had somehow borne witness to something very precious taking place between Dave and Linda. 'Yeah, it felt good to be there with them, and at the same time part of me now wonders whether I should have left the room and let them just be together. Although I don't recall thinking it at the time, it could have become a bit voyeuristic somehow.'

'What was your anxiety, although I'm not sure anxiety is the right word?' Jan asked, sensing how moved Alan was and yet also a sense that he had maybe felt a little awkward. 'No, not anxiety, maybe awkwardness?'

'Not sure what I felt. It just seemed such a tender moment between them. It was a privilege to be there and I am just wondering . . . I'm not sure what I'm wondering, it's something about it all being very fragile and not wanting to kind of damage it I guess. A phrase from a little book came to my mind at the end of the session: "Look for the flower to bloom in the silence that follows the storm: not till then." I had to look up the rest of the passage. There was something very beautiful about what happened between them. I hope it lasts but I fear that it won't.'

'Fear that it won't.' Jan allowed herself to look puzzled. Alan had seemed so positive and yet now he was indicating he had doubts.

'Yes, I don't know, it's alcohol. When alcohol's in the picture you can just never be too sure what is going to happen next.' Alan knew only too well that the kind of experiences both Dave and Linda had been through had left them both vulnerable, and Dave's drinking could easily be triggered. He hoped it wouldn't happen, but he knew the possibility was there.

Jan had the word 'assumption' in her head again and yet it didn't seem to fit. She knew too that where alcohol was concerned things were not always as they seemed, and that achievements were not always maintained. Yet she knew that people did change an alcohol habit and that they could move on. She sensed the stress in Alan as he stood between his conflicting feelings: the hope that what he had witnessed would last and flourish, and that it would help them both to resolve old patterns and drinking behaviours, and the fear that something would go wrong and that the part or parts of Dave's self-structure linked to his heavy drinking would fight back.

She remembered reading that article about the self-concept striking back, how, when you change the part of yourself that you are seeking to change or leave behind, it can seek to reassert itself (Mearns, 1992).

'Alan, I'm just so aware of the tension between holding on to hope and acknowledging fear of further difficulties. You are concerned that Dave's drinking configuration is going to strike back, aren't you?'

'Yes. I don't think we have seen the last of Dave's "lonely me" configuration, and knowing the depth that it can take him to I am fearful.'

'Fearful of?' Jan asked.

'Not sure. If he was depressed I'd be concerned in case it might take him into a suicidal frame of mind. But he hasn't indicated this and I haven't felt any need to ask about suicidal ideation. It simply has not been presented from within his frame of reference, or been a factor that has emerged within my own thoughts and feelings during our interactions. He was quiet in the session initially following his drinking last weekend and into this week, but he did not seem unduly depressed beyond what would be a natural reaction to what had happened. But I know the risk is there if someone really drinks heavily on desperate feelings. I just need to have it in mind, I guess, and I am also aware of a resistance in me to this because I don't want to start carrying that thought into the sessions. I certainly don't want to give him ideas.'

'You think that part of his self-structure, "lonely me", might take him into a suicidal frame of mind?'

'I don't know. I hope not, but I also have to be realistic. It sounds odd talking this way when the last time I saw them they seemed so close, and with so much hope between them to try and make things work and move on. And yet .... ' Alan wasn't sure why he was feeling quite so apprehensive. Was it simply his knowledge and experience of working in this specialty that was triggering this, or was it something genuinely emerging as a product of the therapeutic relationship?

'And yet ... ,' Jan repeated, and a question instantly dropped into her mind. She voiced it. 'Do you routinely feel this way with clients in these kind of situations?'

'No, and this is probably what is concerning me. I haven't anything to support my concerns, but they are very present. I think I need to see if this passes or whether it remains with me. If it remains a nagging concern then I want to say something at the next session, but I want it to be in the context of the interaction that we are having. I need to see whether this is still present next time, and if so, if it is strongly present for me in the session then I will say something. And I will trust myself to say it in a way that expresses my feelings at the time. I don't think a prepared intervention is helpful. I want to say what I need to say in a way that is kind of organic.' Alan felt he would be saying something. It did feel like it was going to persist.

'OK, I am sure you will find the right words in the moment, Alan. Trust your instincts.'

'Yes, this is the part of counselling that some people perceive as being a bit woolly, but we do end up time and time again trusting our instincts, trusting ourselves to be what is helpful within the counselling relationship. I know it is such a part of person-centred working. I can't pre-plan a session, I need it to flow out of the relationship I create with my client as I offer the core conditions. Dave had crap relationships as a child and he's been badly affected. My role is to offer him another experience and a chance to grow, to develop, to discover other ways of being as a result and to offer him the unconditional positive regard he didn't experience in early life.'

'Other ways of being which will become deeply satisfying to him as he recreates his self-structure in response to being in therapeutic relationship with you,' Jan added.

'Yes, and in one sense it is simple, although very difficult and painful in terms of the human experience, and there is the alcohol in the picture which we know can skew people's mood and leave them making destructive choices that they might not have otherwise made.'

'OK, so you will raise the issue of Dave's mood at the next session if your concerns persist?' Jan asked.

'Yes, and I rather feel that I will be raising it as I feel that my concerns are going to persist.' Alan could feel unease in his stomach as he said this. 'I can feel it in here,' he said, patting his belly. 'I felt similar concerns at the end of the session before last concerning the birthday party, and I was right. I need to trust these feelings.'

Jan nodded, she trusted Alan. He was clearly concerned and she knew he would say something and in an appropriate and sensitive way.

She was also aware that something was nagging at her. It was Alan's strong reaction to Linda when he experienced a wish that she would shut up and give Dave some space. She knew she needed to raise this.

'Alan, I'm stuck with something, with wondering what was happening for you when you said you were feeling that you wanted Linda to shut up and give Dave some space. It sounded intense and it feels as though there was a sharp edge to it somehow, or at least that is my wonder. It feels sharp and it is persisting in me.'

Alan thought for a moment. Yes, it had been a sharp moment. And once again Jan had picked something up on the basis that it was worrying at her. He liked her way of working. She trusted her experiences within the supervision relationship and usually when she voiced this kind of nagging discomfort it had value and importance.

'Hmm, yes, that's what I like about you. You don't miss much! I had thought about this and I think I was feeling so close to Dave, so much striving to maintain connection with his inner world plus the history we already had, that I was feeling kind of protective.' Alan had felt Linda was crowding Dave and that Dave needed time to say what he needed to say. He felt he had been protecting Dave's right to say what he wanted to say, but he also acknowledged to himself that he had cut across Linda. 'It has also made me aware of how difficult it can be to work with a couple when you already have a therapeutic relationship with one of them. I want to take this into therapy and look at it more deeply as well. In thinking about it I had a sense that maybe I need to explore this in the context of whether it is a male/female issue.'

'Male/female?' Jan responded, hoping Alan would clarify this further.

'I just wonder if it was a male to male thing that was contributing to my need to maybe protect Dave, and/or whether Linda was hooking some strong feelings in me that were rooted in other experiences. I'm unclear about it at the moment. I just have this sense that I need space in therapy to go into it a little deeper and see what comes up. I want to check out whether my reaction is more than being simply a product of having a closer connection to Dave as a result of our work together over recent weeks.'

'What's you intuitive sense on this, Alan? I think you are right to use therapy to explore it, but I am wondering what you may be sensing within yourself about it.'

> Jan wanted to encourage Alan to listen to his own inner prompting. She would always endeavour to be open to her own reactions and voice anything that she felt needed to be made visible, but she wanted Alan to put into his own words what he was sensing.

'I think it is simply my feelings towards Dave, but I am sufficiently uneasy about it to want to check this out. I think I was in touch with my sense of Dave's vulnerability and he was under pressure and not getting heard. I know I've felt unheard at times and I want to be sure it wasn't hooking this in some way. I want to be clear in myself and about myself. I want space to focus on me. Does that sound reasonable?'

Jan nodded her head. She wanted to encourage Alan to trust his own inner prompting so she responded, 'It seems you have thought this through and have a clear sense of what you want to do. I feel more at ease knowing you were aware of this issue and are taking steps to work on it, or at least clarify it for yourself. It obviously feels important to you to handle it this way.'

'Yes, it does. It seems right to take the emphasis on me to my own therapy, whilst bringing here to supervision more of a focus on Dave and the relationship with him. I know it is hard to separate out sometimes. It all seems a bit artificial at times and I often wonder whether the divide between supervision and personal therapy is actually helpful. Yet at the same time I acknowledge that without some kind of boundary the emphasis in supervision could become overly focused on the counsellor, with little time for clients, and that wouldn't be helpful.'

'So, boundaries are important, and I agree. And your sense is that where the focus becomes too much on the counsellor then the boundary has slipped?' Jan asked, wanting to check she was hearing Alan accurately.

'Yes, and I realise this is an area that in counselling and therapy we are more used to talking about, whilst other professions may not recognise the need for personal work in the same way in order to work effectively with clients. A lot of people I know have line-management supervision, which can offer little or no scope for any personal exploration. And clinical supervision, which can be so focused on diagnosis and how to follow procedures that the relationship gets lost somewhere. Yet for me, so many of the helping professions are about forming relationships with clients, and people are affected by this and do need to explore this. Well, that's what I think anyway. I've strayed back on to my soapbox again! But I do feel strongly that supervision is not well understood. I think people need space to explore their personal reactions to client work, and how they are affected by particular clients and the impact this has on their work with them. And when it becomes a personal issue for the professional involved then some kind of therapeutic work becomes necessary to ensure not only their mental and emotional health, but more importantly that of the client.'

Alan is raising an important point. How do we differentiate management supervision, personal supervision and clinical supervision? There tend to be overlaps but certain professions have developed particular areas of emphasis. Counselling supervision has brought a challenge to clinical and management supervision, demonstrating the importance of some emphasis on the process and personal content of the working relationship.

'You do feel strongly on this, don't you, Alan? I can sense you passion.'

'I have seen too many people burn out through not having appropriate support, partly because it was not offered, but partly because people do not appreciate what could be helpful, or think it is a sign of weakness.' Alan smiled. He felt better getting that off his chest. 'Thanks for listening, Jan. Let's get back to Dave and Linda.'

Jan felt Alan had said what he needed. She agreed he should use personal therapy to explore issues directly present within himself and supervision for relational issues with clients. She agreed with what he had said, as well, about people not understanding the importance and value of supervision. 'OK, so back to Dave and Linda. I am wondering if there is anything else you want to explore about your work with Dave? Are they coming back as a couple?'

'They wanted to keep it open for a future time, but for now Dave will continue to come weekly. That is what they wanted and it felt right. Maybe Linda may decide to seek some kind of counselling to help her make sense of her past and how it has affected her, but at the moment she is not looking for this. She may change. It must have been a powerful experience for her in that last session. I will continue to work with Dave, be there for him as he . . . well, who knows where it will take him. But I was encouraged by that sense of calm and OKness he found during that pit experience. And the fact that I was drawn to that spiritual passage at the end of the last session. There's something deep to Dave. Whilst I am concerned for his well-being, I also have a sense that somehow he will be OK. I hope I'm right.'

'Maybe it is important to acknowledge that depth that you sense as well.'

'You know I see life as a bit of a journey down a river, or rather we are the river. Sometimes it is smooth, we are smooth; sometimes it, and we, are a raging torrent. Sometimes there are rapids and waterfalls. Dave is going through some rapids, but there is a stillness or *calmness*, to use his word. Yet it is not an aspect of himself he is familiar with. But he glimpsed it in that session and I am sure it has made a deep impression. I know it did. It's like he has sensed a possibility within himself and I don't think it will go away. I often see clients yearning for some kind of peace, but they provoke chaos because that is what they have been conditioned into from an early age. They often have a dim sense of wanting change, but of not being sure exactly what they want. I think Dave has sensed something in himself that is essentially calm and maybe that will become a more present aspect of his nature in the future.'

How many times had he, Alan, heard clients say how they yearned for some peace, that they were getting too old for the drinking, or they just wanted to settle down, but couldn't get away from old habits. He recognised the conflicts within Dave, the different 'voices' from the different elements within his self-structure. They were all part of Dave but he knew that for the drinking to be brought under control, Dave would have to recreate his sense of self, rebalance the elements that made him who he was and probably introduce some new ones. These could not be forced. It was for them to develop within Dave in response to the experience of being in a warm and unconditionally accepting relationship, as he came to know himself more clearly in response to communicated and heard empathic responses and the experience of entering into a therapeutic relationship with someone seeking to be congruent.

Summary

Alan brings his experiences of working with Dave in the past three sessions to Jan, who picks up on the possibility that his own recent history may be impacting on his work in relation to Dave's previous 'pit' experience. Alan plans to explore this in personal therapy. The theme of assumptions is raised and explored, along with whether Dave is carrying any suicidal potential, and when this might be raised by Alan. Alan also recognises his need to take his possible overprotectiveness towards Dave into personal therapy. The presence of Alan's concern for Dave and his confidence that he will be OK are highlighted.

Points for discussion

- Is it possible that Jan and Alan should have explored assumptions further here? Maybe an assumption was being made by them that Dave was not likely to enter into a suicidal state.
- How would you define and differentiate counselling, management and clinical supervision?
- Where do you distinguish supervision issues from personal therapy issues?
- How would you define intuition and what role does it have in counselling?
- What is the theoretical basis for raising issues (such as Dave's mood) only when they are present in the 'here and now' of the therapeutic relationship?

Wider issues

- Issues about the relationship we have with clients and the assumptions that we make have applications for all the helping professions.
- The need for reflection on practice promotes greater self-awareness and minimises the risk of content within the helping professional's self-structure reducing the effectiveness of what they are offering the client.

Wednesday morning, 29 November

Dave arrived on time, and looked positive. 'Hi Alan, things are feeling good again. A good week.' Dave's eye contact was much steadier, Alan thought. Interesting that it had made such an impact on him. He had not forgotten the supervision discussion around concern for Dave's mood and suicidal potential, but it did not feel pressing, and to introduce it would take Dave away from his current focus. He let it go and stayed with what Dave had said and kept his response simple to allow Dave to continue.

'Feeling good.'

'Yeah, I've got back in control again, and have had some long talks with Linda. You know, I really was shocked by what she said last week. I just had no idea what she had gone through and how much she was affected by my going out to the pub. What she went through as a child. I know how it feels to have a tough time, but at least there weren't feelings of threat in the atmosphere. I mean, I was just, well, I wasn't physically hurt. I was just left to get on with it.'

Alan realised he could have paraphrased what Dave had just said, but he could sense that Dave was moving and rather than stop him to show him that he had heard him completely, he felt it best to simply feed back the last thing said. Dave was journeying and there was no point in recounting the whole journey back to him. Maybe that might be learned in counselling skills, but not in therapeutic counselling. The counsellor has to be empathic not only to what is being said, but to how it is being said and to the client's process.

'Just left to get on with it,' Alan responded.

'Yes, and I survived. OK, it affected me. I know that now – only too well – but I survived, yeah, and I'm going to move on.' Dave felt strong, he felt like a survivor but he also realised that for him what he had survived did not feel as bad as what he felt Linda had gone through.

'You survived, Dave, and now you are going to move on, that's it?'

'Sure am. I've done really well this week. I'm back off the lunch-time drinking again and have had some dry evenings as well. Not been easy, mind you. Kept myself occupied.' Dave was feeling really pleased. He felt that the session before with Linda had really had a profound effect on him. He had felt deeply touched by what had happened, by what Linda had talked about. He somehow felt more sensitive. He felt more able to hear her pain in some way. This was kind of new to him, to feel this, well actually to feel at all. He had realised how little he did feel day to day, except for those times when he was overwhelmed by feelings, like loneliness or feeling left out.

Alan felt good that Dave had done so well. He could feel himself smiling. Should he allow himself to show that he felt good, or should he remain impartial? Alan's philosophy was that as a therapist he was first of all a person with human thoughts, feelings and reactions. He was seeking to be in a 'person-to-person' therapeutic relationship. (He had always thought the 'person-to-person' summed it up and was inspired by the journal that he read of that name – *see* useful contacts list on page 186.) He wanted to bring as much as he could of himself into therapeutic relationships with his clients. *Transparency*, there's a way of being to achieve. He knew how important but also how hard it was – one of the great challenges of the discipline of person-centred counselling, he thought to himself, but so releasing, so liberating both for the therapist and for the client when it is present. Alan also recognised how challenging it could be for the client who was struggling with incongruence, who felt unable to disclose aspects of him or herself or behaviours that were known but which carried some degree of shame or discomfort.

'You look really pleased, and I feel really pleased. Couldn't have been easy, as you say.' Alan tried to be transparent with his feelings.
'No, not easy at all,' Dave replied. 'That first evening after we saw you, well, after putting the children to bed we both sat and talked. We were both in tears again at times, but it felt so good to share, to listen, to feel heard, to, I don't know, somehow begin to get real with each other. We'd both been carrying secrets around for years, stuff we hadn't talked of, fears we both had. I couldn't have done that a few months back.'
'Couldn't have talked and listened like that?' Alan responded with a hint of questioning in his voice.
'Just wouldn't have happened, wouldn't have been interested. If I had been there I would have been more interested in thinking about when I was going out for a drink. And Linda wouldn't have said anything. She never talked about that part of her childhood, why should she, I wouldn't have listened any more than she probably wouldn't have listened to me, or I guess that's how it would have been. I suppose I don't know. It never really happened. We were in a rut, but now we're out of it. God it's good to talk, and even better to feel heard.

You've taught me that as well, Alan. You were the one that started listening to me, who accepted me. That made a profound impact on me, though I wasn't aware of it at the time. I didn't really know what to make of all this.'

Alan felt good and he was sufficiently self-aware to recognise within himself a sense that whilst he hoped Dave had established a change that he could build on and grow from, he was also aware that it was still early days and Dave had some deep-seated sensitivities that could arise and trigger further drinking episodes. He decided to stay in Dave's frame of reference whilst being prepared to voice his inner feelings should they persist.

'Hmmm. You had come along here and were being affected in ways that you really didn't appreciate at the time, but which you can now see were profound,' Alan responded.

'Yeah. I don't think I need to see you any more. I mean, it's under control now. Linda and I are talking and I feel that I'm OK. It's been such a good week. What do you think?' Alan was aware that Dave was looking at him, expecting an answer, and no doubt an agreement. Well, he didn't feel comfortable with this and he wanted to voice this and acknowledge Dave's feelings as well.

'You want to know what *I* think?' he replied, in a sense double-checking that this was what Dave really wanted.

'Yeah, I mean, you must see that I'm doing well.'

'I do, and I am aware of just how positive you are feeling about it. No hint of concern?'

'No, I'm feeling good.' Dave was feeling good, but he wanted to know what Alan thought though. He wanted Alan to agree that he was OK now, that he could get on with his life and not have to think of himself as having a drink problem. He wanted Alan to support him in his wanting to believe that he was 'cured'. Of course, deep down Dave knew that he wasn't really free of the drinking problem, but he had had enough of the discomfort around it . He wanted to get on, and he needed Alan to support him in this. 'So what do you think?'

Meanwhile, Alan was aware that he really did have reservations about Dave stopping. He sensed this was a critical time in the therapeutic relationship and in Dave's own process of coming to terms with having a drink problem. 'What do I think? I really hear your confidence Dave, I really do, and I also want to be honest with you because I respect you, and I want to be real with you. I want to believe that you are free of the problem, and maybe you are in terms of the drinking, maybe you are, I don't know. But are you free of the sensitivities that have triggered you into drinking? Are you 100 per cent sure that you are going to be able to sustain control?'

Alan said the last sentence very slowly. He wanted his words to really sink in for Dave. He knew that he did not feel at all at ease with the idea that Dave was OK, yet he didn't want to undermine Dave. He wanted to give Dave the chance to evaluate his own thoughts and feelings about his drinking. If Dave said he was 100 per cent sure, he would be concerned that he was overconfident or maybe wanting to avoid further counselling. If he wasn't 100 per cent he felt this to be more realistic, and it could open up the opportunity of exploring what was making him unsure so that the risk of a relapse might be minimised. Alan felt that if he could help Dave acknowledge or connect with his doubts then it would also help him towards a more complete appreciation of his situation, and maybe then Dave's tendency towards growth, towards greater completeness in himself, would urge him to want to address these doubts. Whilst he didn't want to sit there with a head full of goals for Dave, he also needed to be realistic. Alan waited for Dave to respond.

'No, I can't be 100 per cent sure. I'd be foolish to believe that,' was Dave's response. Alan felt relief. He, Dave, was stepping back into a realistic perspective. 'But I feel I am ready to give it a go on my own. I know what I need to do. I'm getting good support at home.'

'OK Dave, I hear you, and I want to work with you to be sure that we minimise the risk of further problems occurring. So what I am sitting here wondering is what is it that stops you being 100 per cent sure?'

Dave was silent. He was looking down and in himself he was feeling very uncertain. He could feel waves of fear flowing through him, but he really did not want to show them. He wanted to be strong. He wanted to move on. He didn't want to go back and remember his past. Yet the feelings of fear would not go away. He hadn't felt fear like this for years. He lost all track of time as he sat there. Then a memory bubbled into his thinking, originating out of those early days as a teenager, wanting to be part of the group, but feeling always on the outside looking in. And the girls never wanted to know him. Trying to talk to them was so scary. He remembered how he used to panic. He didn't want to go back there again, but he was there. He looked up. He could feel the tension in his stomach and his throat was going dry. He tried to hide his anxieties by smiling, but it was a weak smile and he knew it. And he knew Alan would see through it. This was not going to be easy, but he began to find the words and slowly he revealed the fears that were inside him.

'I'm scared of getting caught up in my past. I'm scared of re-experiencing some of those early feelings. I'm scared of everything falling apart and I don't want to feel scared any more.'

'Scared of so many things,' Alan replied, wanting to keep it open so Dave could take it wherever he needed. 'And you don't want to feel scared any more.'

Dave was shaking his head. 'No.' He was taking deep breaths and blowing the air out. 'No, I fucking don't. I've had enough of all these feelings. I've had enough of being me.' The words exploded out of Dave's mouth and he slammed his fist down on the arm of the chair, looking at Alan, his jaw set, his teeth gritted. 'I've had enough of being me, of being scared, of being lonely, of being all the things we have talked about. I want a normal life. I want everything to settle down. I want to find some peace. Is that too much to ask?'

'Makes you fucking angry, Dave. Had enough of what you feel and you want some peace, yeah?'

'Too fucking right.' Dave paused. He wasn't sure what to say next. He had been surprised himself by his outburst. 'I don't know, I want to believe I'm OK, I really do. But there is part of me that doubts whether I am. It has been a good week, and I'm scared of losing it, and that fear is setting off memories of older fears. Oh God, what a mess. I came in here feeling so good, so positive. Now look at me.' Dave stopped speaking and put his head in his hands.

Alan could feel his compassion for Dave and he put out his hand to touch Dave on the arm. It was an instinctive reaction, not thought through, the kind of response he had learned to trust. He knew if he was to be effective with a client he had to be wholly present and bring his whole nature into the relationship. He had to trust prompting from within his own organism. He wanted to reach out to Dave in his inner world of fear. Dave looked up and nodded. He didn't pull his arm away.

'Shit, it's hard in here,' Dave spoke softly and looked up at the ceiling, tears in his eyes. 'I never believed I had so many feelings. I feel like I'm on a roller coaster, or something.' He blew out his breath, 'Oh dear.' Then breathed in deeply again, the air filling his lungs, and then he let it go again, shaking his head.

'So hard to be you,' Alan responded, again a mixture of affirmation and questioning, wanting to allow Dave to feel that he, Alan, was hearing how hard it was.

'Yeah.' Dave could feel he was beginning to settle down again.

Alan stayed silent. He was still holding Dave's arm and it felt comfortable. He didn't want to withdraw it as it seemed OK and he didn't want Dave to feel that he was backing away. The silence continued.

When to reach out and touch someone, or when to withdraw that contact, is often a challenge for counsellors. Alan is trusting his inner prompting, a spontaneous human response. If we cannot bring our humanity into the counselling room then we surely lose something that is extremely precious and that can be powerfully therapeutic.

Alan was experiencing a tremendous sense of just how hard it was for Dave. 'So hard to be Dave,' he said quietly and waited.

'I find it hard to feel at ease with myself sometimes, well, a lot of the time actually.' Dave hadn't planned to be in touch with these feelings, but they were very present for him now. He heard Alan's empathic response, 'Hard to feel at ease with yourself not just sometimes, but a lot of the time.'

Dave could feel a gentle kind of turmoil inside himself, a sort of disorientation. His heart was thumping now and he could feel a cold sweat coming on. He heard himself say something that sort of shocked him, as it wasn't something he had thought about saying. The words were suddenly there, coming out of his mouth. 'I don't know who I am.'

Alan heard Dave utter those words and saw the shock on his face. He felt he could do nothing other than hold that phrase for Dave, hold it gently and await a response. He repeated Dave's words slowly and deliberately, 'I don't know who I am.'

Dave could feel himself shaking his head yet he seemed to be empty of thought. He just sat, feeling immobile. Ages seemed to pass by. He breathed deeply and felt himself frowning. He looked up at Alan. 'I want to know who I am. I want to find the real Dave. I want to get rid of all the crap I've accumulated. I want to get free of all the fears. I want to . . . .' His words trailed off into silence and he bit his lip.

Alan could sense that there were unspoken words though he did not know what they were. He reflected back Dave's final three words in the hope that Dave might continue and finish what he was in the process of saying, 'I want to . . . .'

Dave took another deep breath. 'I was going to say, "I want to live", but that seemed kind of stupid. I mean, I am alive, but there is something more to me. I know it. But all this crap is in the way. All these insecurities.'

'You want to live but there is a lot of crap getting in the way of that happening, is that how it is?' Alan phrased it as a question to hold Dave and to create an opportunity to clarify for himself that he had heard right. Dave was silent. Alan had sensed the desperation in Dave's voice. He decided to name this and simply said, in a soft voice, 'Desperately wanting to live . . . .'

'There has to be more to life than going down the pub every night. I've been doing it for so long. I've got so used to it. And then it all gets over the top. Once I start drinking I can't seem to stop. I don't want to stop. It's like a brake is taken off, and it's downhill all the way into oblivion. I can't keep doing it. But I'm scared of life without it.'

'Scared of life without it, and scared of not being able to stop the plunge into oblivion.'

Dave lapsed back into silence again. Minutes passed. He was realising something he knew he had been pushing aside, not wanting to face. He knew it was this that was behind his wanting to end the counselling. Like so many others he knew now he had been looking for an excuse to stop getting help and to carry on drinking, yet he also didn't want this as well. It felt so crazy. He could feel the fear again, and now he knew what it was, it scared the hell out of him. 'I'm scared of finding out that I can't pull out of the dive.' He looked up at Alan straight into his eyes.

It was a moment of deep contact. Alan met Dave's eyes and the two sat silently. Alan felt tremendous compassion for Dave, for his uniqueness as a person and the tremendous personal struggle he was encountering in his life. He saw the desperation, the pleading in Dave's eyes. It was a moment when the distance between them melted away and neither Dave nor Alan felt separate from each other. There was a profound coming together in that moment, a moment that seemed to step out of time in some inexplicable way, yet each seemed so alert to everything going on within themselves. Somehow, and this seemed a strange paradox, whilst he felt the depth of connection with Dave he also felt a sharper, clearer sense of his and Dave's own uniqueness as persons. A kind of moment of distinction and connection that defied human logic, but was nevertheless being experienced.

After some minutes it began to fade for Alan and it was he who spoke first having noticed Dave's facial expression change and a slight smile appear on his face. He was aware of experiencing a deep yearning to help Dave pull back from what he feared would happen, yet he also knew that he must trust Dave's own inner process. He knew he must be ready to offer Dave companionship wherever he went within his experience of himself. Yet he also wanted to offer a sense of what he felt about the depth of Dave's fear and despair.

'Scary, scary place, and I kind of see a bit of a smile on your lips as well,' were the words that came out of his mouth. He really did not know what else to say. This was the overwhelming impression that he had had of Dave's world from his experience of being with Dave in those last few minutes and of what he was now seeing on Dave's face.

Dave nodded, 'Yeah,' and blew out a breath. 'Now I know what I'm up against.'

Alan was aware that whilst he had heard Dave's words, he wasn't at all sure what he was meaning. He had sensed the scariness, but not what it was that was scary. He frowned and asked, 'You are now sure what you are up against?'

'Fear. Fear of failure, fear of not being strong enough, fear of losing myself. And I know this sounds strange but I have this sense that I have to lose myself to find myself. Does that make any sense?'

Alan felt himself smile for he did have an understanding of what Dave was saying although he recognised that his understanding may not be what Dave meant, so he needed to be careful to stay clearly with what Dave was wanting to communicate. 'You have to lose something of yourself in order to find some other aspect of yourself, or are you saying you have a sense that you have to lose your whole self in order to find a new whole self?'

'I don't know, but something has to go before I can become something else. And that's, well, I want to say frightening but I am also aware that it also feels exciting too. That's new. But there is an excitement around as well.'

'So in part you are frightened, but also excited, and the excitement is a new experience?' Again Alan phrased it as a question, to clarify that he was hearing correctly what Dave was wanting to communicate.

Empathic responses voiced as questions can have this useful dual role of allowing the client to hear what they have said but in a way that can facilitate their own self-questioning, which can lead to clarity and a deeper, more precise experience of what is present.

'Yeah, it feels exciting to feel that something new is possible, even though I'm not sure what that means.' Dave was really surprised by this sense of increasing excitement. A little while ago he was in utter fear and despair, now he was almost on a high – well, on the way up anyway.

Alan had a phrase come into his head and he wondered whether he was just going to end up sounding as if he was trying to be clever, but the phrase wasn't something he had deliberately formulated, it was just there in his head. He voiced it. 'Seems like you've just pulled out of a nose dive.'

Dave smiled grimly and shook his head, 'And I didn't have to try, it just happened. What is this all about? What did I say a little while back, "feels like I'm on a roller coaster". Couldn't have been more true. One minute I seemed to be looking down this great drop and the next I was somehow in a different place.'

'In a different place?' Alan asked enquiringly.

'Yeah. And I don't know what that was about. I really don't.' Dave shook his head. 'Something else to go away and think about.'

Alan nodded his head. He had glanced at the clock and was aware that time was running out. It felt as though Dave was in a sense rounding off his journey within the session. The depth had definitely lifted. Alan wondered how Dave would want to use the rest of the time. 'We've only got a few more minutes, Dave. I'm wondering how you want to use them.'

'I don't know. I feel as though I have just been on one hell of a journey and it will take a while for me to regain my focus.'

'You need to ground yourself a bit, get back into focus before moving back outside. Do you want to stay around for a while, have a cup of tea just to give yourself a little more time?'

Alan was aware how disorientating counselling can be. He wanted Dave to take the time he needed to regain his focus. In his experience, therapy could leave you like plucked cotton wool, all loose and wispy round the edges and in need of time to re-compact itself. Of course, the magic was that one never re-compacted in quite the same way. Sometimes you could name the difference; at other times it was subtle and you could be quite unaware of it until some time later when you suddenly found yourself behaving or reacting differently to a familiar situation.

'Yeah, I think I will, and just sit quietly for a few minutes.' Dave somehow knew something significant had happened but he was not really clear exactly what.

'You can use this room. It's free for the next 15 minutes or so. I'll get some tea.' Alan did not want Dave going back into the waiting area. He wanted him to have his own space to sit quietly and reflect.

The session ended and after a period of reflection Dave felt ready to head off back to work. He didn't really know what had happened, but he knew he felt different somehow. It was like he knew what he was up against but he didn't as well. He had a sense of the profound nature of the challenge before him yet he couldn't really grasp its implications. He knew, though, that somehow life would never be the same. He could remember the fear and he sensed the excitement as well.

Yet he also knew he was neither of these feelings for he was somehow observing them both. There was that strange sense of being transported to some other place in himself that he could not define. He felt strong, but a different strong to how he had thought he felt at the start of the session.

Alan reflected back on that sense of uniqueness and connection with Dave. He recalled a comment written by Brian Thorne: 'It seems as if for a space, however brief, two human beings are fully alive because they have given themselves and each other permission to risk being fully alive. At such a moment I have no hesitation in saying that my client and I are caught up in a stream of love' (Thorne, 1985, p.9). Love, Alan mused. A word not often used in therapy yet was it not more than anything else the secret of healthy relationship? Yet there were so many forms of love, and it could be so selfish and damaging as well as unconditional and healing. He smiled, for he remembered a book in which, in the first printing, 'core conditions' had been misprinted as 'love conditions' (Frances and Bryant-Jefferies, 1998). Perhaps a deep truth had been accidentally revealed in that 'error'!

Summary

Dave attends feeling good and feeling he is ready to move on. Alan is unsure and asks him if he is 100 per cent certain. Dave is not and it triggers him into an angry outburst, and of wanting to feel normal. Alan reaches out to Dave. A moment of deep contact is experienced between Dave and Alan. Dave goes into himself and faces his fears, seeing them clearly and feeling as though he is at risk of plunging into them. He feels fear and excitement yet, rather than plunge into them, feels as though he is transported within himself to another place. He knows he has changed but is unsure what has happened.

Points for discussion

- Alan challenged Dave's certainty around his control of his alcohol use out of his own sense of unease. Should all challenges only be expressions of congruent experiencing?
- When is physical contact with a client appropriate? How comfortable are you with this form of response?
- What was happening to Dave as he encountered his fears and how might the other place that he found himself in be explained or described?
- Imagine that Dave had not pulled out of the dive and had been overwhelmed by a feeling of fear along the lines that he indicated. How, as a counsellor, would you react when faced with this?
- What would you do, and how would you feel, if such a nose dive occurred right at the end of the session?

Wider focus

- The topic of physical contact with clients needs to be thought through within all helping professions.
- Clients can enter into very scary places and feel overwhelmed. Often we need to have faced our own fears in order to be a companion to another who is encountering their own fears.

Wednesday morning, 6 December

Dave arrived 15 minutes late. Alan had been wondering whether Dave might have slipped back into drinking and that something had happened, or that he might have felt ashamed to come because of it. Yet he also wanted to hold on to an optimistic outlook. So he felt genuinely pleased when Dave arrived. Dave had come direct from home but had got caught in traffic and hadn't got his mobile phone with him. He explained to Alan what had happened.

'Still feeling good, Alan, and I've really cut back now. I just don't feel an urge to drink. It's as though that part of me has gone, or at least lost its grip on me.' Dave had sat down and was looking at Alan with a smile on his face. He certainly looked a better colour to Alan, and he seemed much more alert.

'Still drinking a little but not feeling any urge to drink at all now?' was Alan's response, said with an awareness that it contained the in-built contradiction that Dave had voiced. If he had no urge to drink, why was he still drinking?

'No, well, apart from the odd can in the evenings, that 5% lager, but not every evening. I've got into some work around the house in the evenings and it really is doing me some good. Linda is pleased as well. Some of the jobs have been around for a long time, just haven't got down to them. Now I'm getting a good sense of achievement. But there is still a lot more to do. But that is good.'

'So, it feels like a real achievement. And whilst I want to acknowledge that, I also want to say that I am stuck with wondering about the odd can when you are not experiencing an urge to drink. Clearly it doesn't seem to be a problem to you . . . .' Alan was aware that the contradiction in not feeling an urge to drink yet choosing to drink was still with him.

'No, not a problem, but yes it feels different now. I can honestly take it or leave it. Let's see, yesterday was dry, so was Monday. I had a couple of cans Sunday afternoon watching TV, a couple Saturday evening and a couple Friday evening. Thursday and Wednesday of last week were dry.'

'Sounds like a big change,' Alan acknowledged. 'Six cans in the past week, what's that, around 12 units for 5% strength.'

'And there is no doubt I do feel better for it. I just feel so much clearer, more motivated. Something is definitely different in me.'

'So, feeling better, clearer, more motivated. Something has changed in you.' Alan kept to a simple empathic reflection.

'Yeah, I want to explore this today and I want to discuss what to do now about my level of drinking.'

Alan did not want to push Dave in one direction or the other. He felt Dave would know what was most important to him, so he voiced this: 'So, which direction do you want to go in?'

Dave sat and thought for a few moments. 'It seems odd really. Last week I wanted to stop, thinking I had control, but then realised how little control I had and how I was fearful of failure. This week I feel more genuinely confident, yet want to make more sense of my drinking. I want to look at the drinking pattern. Although it doesn't feel like a problem, I am aware that Christmas isn't too far away and I really need to think it through. I mean, I think I'll be OK, but it isn't going to be easy even though at the moment I do feel in control. And I was thinking back to last week, to wanting to end the sessions, and I realise just how mistaken I was. I need this contact, it helps me to keep my focus.'

'So the sessions help you to focus. And I'm wondering what aspect of Christmas is troubling you?'

Alan was well aware that Christmas was a difficult time for drinkers who were trying to maintain control. It had strong drinking associations for many people, and was a time when people could relapse and go on to a lengthy binge. People are often put under pressure to drink. There would be more parties and opportunities to drink at Christmas and many people with drinking problems could have bad memories associated with that time of year. Families get together and past tensions and difficulties can re-emerge, triggering people into 'configurations of self' associated with past experiences which in turn may themselves be drinking triggers.

'It's just that I've never really had a Christmas when I have not been drunk much of the time. It will be a new experience and it is hard to imagine. I want to be in control. I want to be able to have a few drinks, but not let it get out of control.' Dave knew there was likely to be a lot of socialising and parties, and he wasn't too sure how he would cope sober.

Alan responded, aware that coming through the Christmas and New Year period was going to be a big achievement for Dave, if he could make it. 'So, a sober Christmas is hard to imagine with all the socialising, parties, etc. You plan to have a few drinks but don't want to lose control, is that right?'

'Yeah. I guess I'm wondering whether I need to avoid some of the parties, or what to do. I don't want to not have a good time, but I don't want to take risks either. I feel I'll be OK, but ... ,' Dave shrugged his shoulders.

Alan appreciated what he meant. It was all very uncertain and with the best will in the world things could slide. Alan could feel an urge to make suggestions. He wanted to try to help Dave come to his own conclusions, though, rather than pitch in with a list of suggestions. How many times had this come up with clients. He had enough ideas to write a book: looking for alternative activities, planning what to say to people to avoid being pushed into drinking, thinking through alternative drinks. So many ideas were good, but they generally only worked if the person themself really wanted them to, and they really owned the ideas as well. He hoped Dave would formulate his own strategy, thereby helping him to continue to build up his 'internal locus of evaluation', as Rogers (1961, p.354) termed it. He did not want to undermine this by being too 'expert' on the situation. Yet if Dave really was stuck for ideas, and really did want some suggestions, then he would at least try to trigger a brainstorming session with an idea or two to help Dave to realise that he had options and choices.

'So what do you think will help you, Dave?' Alan asked, genuinely wanting to hear what Dave had already thought through.

'Well, we usually go to the local pub for Christmas Eve, and now I'm not going there so much, well hardly ever, I'm not sure whether or not to go. I've always drunk heavily there, and I want to avoid that. But I don't really want to miss out.'

'Miss out?' Alan asked, wanting to clarify what Dave meant by this.

'Well, you know, everyone's out for a laugh and it's a great time. Wouldn't want to miss it really.'

'OK, so it has been a good experience in the past and you don't want to miss out on that this Christmas.' After a pause Alan added, in response to how he had heard Dave speak, 'Not missing out on the Christmas Eve experience seems incredibly important to you.'

'Well, yes, I suppose, but not if it messes up Christmas. Oh, I don't know. I'm so confused. I don't know if it is a good idea to drink at all, and yet I do want to feel able to have a few drinks. I just want to keep it under control.' Dave was feeling uncomfortable. He knew Christmas was a risky time, but the idea of a dry Christmas just did not have much appeal.

'Should you go for a dry Christmas, or should you try for planned and controlled drinking? Confusing,' was Alan's response, communicating Dave's dilemma back to him and giving him time to ponder on these words.

'I want to enjoy it but I don't want to mess up. I don't want to put myself at risk. I need to distance myself from temptation, don't I?' he asked, looking at Alan, who nodded and responded.

'Need to distance yourself from temptation,' Alan replied.

'Yeah. Easy to say. How to do it though?'

'How do you think you can do that then?' Alan responded with a direct question rather than a questioning reflection. It had the effect of focusing Dave on solutions rather than the question itself.

'I need to avoid places where alcohol is very available and there is a lot of drinking. I really don't think I can trust myself. I'm going to have to turn down some of the invites this year. I'm not going to feel good about it, but I don't see any other way.' Dave could feel himself sighing but he knew he was right. It was going to have to be a dry, or near-dry, Christmas. He couldn't risk sliding back into the old pattern. 'OK, I'm going to have to think of some other things to do. I guess the kids will be up for a few things and maybe I need to focus more on them.'

'So go for dry and get more involved with the children.' Alan felt a sense of this being a great idea but at the moment that was all it was. How was it to be achieved? He let the concern remain within him and waited for Dave to respond.

'Yeah, and I'll avoid the office party this year. I don't need to be there. And maybe we'll go out if the weather's OK, get down to the coast or something. I need to talk to Linda. We've got to go to her mother's on Boxing Day. She doesn't drink much so if we don't take anything, then there won't be much opportunity.'

Alan was aware the concern was not moving. He wanted to acknowledge Dave's ideas and comment on his feelings. 'These sound like good ideas, Dave. What about the other days? I am aware of wondering how you are going to reduce the risk of drinking then.'

'Not sure. It is still a few weeks away. Maybe I'll have a chat with Linda and see what we can organise. Yeah, I'm sure we'll come up with some ideas. We have got time to make a few plans.'

'Sounds positive. I feel it is important to think these things through. Christmas can be a tough time for someone trying to control alcohol use, or remain dry, possibly for the first time. So, you'll have a chat with Linda and see what ideas you come up with together.'

Silence followed and Alan felt he wanted to check with Dave that he had said all he wanted to at this time about Christmas. 'So, do you feel you have explored this enough for the moment? And I am aware you said earlier that you also wanted to explore your current drinking pattern, and the sense of something having changed within you.'

'Yeah, I have time to think through Christmas. It feels good to have aired it, and that you have taken my concerns seriously. I knew I needed to at least begin to talk it through. So thanks for that. As for my drinking pattern, currently I'm drinking, what, about eight cans a week, with dry days. Do you think I should stick at that or should I try to reduce further?' Dave was aware that he rather liked those evening cans, and they didn't seem a problem.

'And it feels OK to you?' Alan responded.

'I think so. But you hear people say that you have to stop to really get over an alcohol problem. But I don't feel I need to stop. I'm not feeling tempted to drink every day. I've broken that habit. I feel more in control.'

'So you feel more in control and I am aware of wondering how much you feel you are in control of the decision to have a couple of cans. Could you say "no" on an evening when you had planned to have a drink? Or do you think you would justify it to yourself somehow and still have the cans?' Alan noticed that Dave was smiling.

Alan knew he had moved out of Dave's frame of reference, but he really wanted to help Dave clarify what he meant by feeling in control. Just how much control did he have? He felt it important to help Dave with this. He knew how easily people could fool themselves into believing they had control when in reality they did not. Dave clearly wanted to address his alcohol use and Alan felt it would be unprofessional and somewhat unhelpful to not introduce this question. It was easy to say no on the days when you did not feel like a drink, but the days when you did were another matter entirely.

Dave knew he was smiling because he knew that it was a damned good question Alan had raised. Was he really in control? He liked to think he was, but was he? 'Am I in control of my choice to have a couple of cans? I really want to say yes, but I have this sneaky feeling that the truth is no. How can I be sure? I do want to be in control. I don't want those cans controlling me. Yet I enjoy a drink and don't want to lose that enjoyment either.'

'So, you want to gain a sense of enjoyment which you currently get through a couple of cans, but you don't want to be at risk of losing control.' Alan was aware how so many drinkers had a threshold. They could drink a certain amount and maybe be OK, but over a certain limit and rational thinking was suppressed and the choice to continue drinking becomes the most reasonable thing in the world.

'I guess I'm caught between being curious about what this enjoyment actually is, and not wanting to take you away from the notion of wanting to be in control.'

'I enjoy the relaxation, that kind of loosened-up feeling. A couple of cans helps me unwind.'

Alan felt a response building up inside himself, 'Helps you relax, like nothing else'. The 'like nothing else' was irresistible to say. He smiled inwardly, knowing that whilst this was coming from his experience of working with drinkers, he had a good sense that this was going to be in line with Dave's experience as well.

When working with a particular client group certain common experiences do emerge. Sometimes you have a sense of how it is for the client in front of you not because of what they have said, but because of the experience of other people with similar problems. Voicing what you know is not what one might call 'responsive empathy', in the sense of being empathic in response to what a client has communicated themselves, but is more of a 'generalised empathy' that is highly likely to have relevance to the client.

'Like nothing else . . . .' Dave thought about this and Alan left him with his thoughts. He could sense by Dave's frown and concentrated expression that it was a working silence. 'But there have to be other ways to relax. I mean, is that what it has come to? I can only feel good after a few cans?' Dave was feeling somewhat angry with himself. And he could feel that little voice justifying how it was OK to have a couple of cans, that it wasn't a problem, and much less than many people drink.

'You look a bit angry about it. Brings up some strong feelings?' Alan heard the anger but he wanted to keep it open for other feelings to maybe emerge as well.

'Yeah, well, I was just thinking that two cans isn't much, and yet I want to feel in control. Let me stick at this pattern for a week or two and see how it goes. I want to get a sense of how much control I actually have here. I'll track it on the drinking diaries and keep a tab on my feelings and what's going on around the drinking.'

'So what you are saying is that you'd like to have a period maintaining this change, to get accustomed to it, before considering further change.'

'Yeah,' Dave replied.

This is the classic 'cycle of change' maintenance phase, Alan thought, and as ever with maintenance you could never be sure how long it would be before it was finally established as a new pattern or behaviour. After how long does change become sustainable change? Had Dave changed enough in himself to sustain a much reduced level of alcohol intake?

Thinking of it in terms of this model (Prochaska and DiClemente, 1982) also brought Alan's thoughts to relapse as well. What if Dave relapsed? Should he introduce some relapse prevention ideas? He didn't want to move out of Dave's frame of reference; he wanted to maintain his client-centred focus and yet the more he sat with it the more it felt important to say something. He wanted Dave to achieve his goal of sustaining a reduced level of alcohol intake. Yet he also knew he needed to be transparent and not hide what were, in one sense, concerns yet were also the product of his general experience.

'I'm wondering if there is anything coming up that you think might put this maintained change at risk.' Alan wanted to own his feelings. He didn't think a comment like, 'So, what if you relapse?' was particularly helpful. He wanted his experiencing of being in relationship with Dave to be reflected in what he said, and he genuinely was wondering what might put Dave's new drinking pattern at risk.

Dave thought for a while. The next couple of weeks seemed fairly normal and like the last one. He was working during the week, and it was going to be a busy week with the training days he had to attend and the meeting on Wednesday that meant he wouldn't be able to get to see Alan. It would be the usual routine at home. Weekends he hadn't really got anything planned, although he wanted to carry on with some decorating and a few DIY jobs that needed attending to. Linda was away at her mother's on Saturday week with the kids. He was going to watch football in the afternoon at home, put his feet up, relax a little, probably get a take-away in the evening for when Linda came back. All seemed fairly normal. 'No, nothing much happening that seems like a problem to me. But it is a busy week at work and I think I'm not going to be able to get to see you. I'll need an appointment for the following week. Is that OK?'

Alan felt OK. He was realistic. People had other priorities sometimes. Dave seemed fairly stable and was indicating his sense that nothing difficult was expected in the next couple of weeks. He wanted to double-check with Dave, though. 'If you need to be at work then that's where you need to be. You know where I am, though. If something does come up and it is leaving you feeling at risk of drinking more than you are planning, please give me a call. And you have the helpline numbers as well for weekends, just in case. Do you feel OK about two weeks to the next appointment?'

'Yes, I feel positive, but I don't feel complacent any more. I think I have a more realistic sense of what I am up against. Not feeling complacent seems to be part of that change I am experiencing. I'm not experiencing an urge to drink heavily and I am pleased about that.'

'So, you feel more realistic, less complacent. More in touch with the reality of the situation. You are not feeling a strong urge to drink heavily or problematically. And I am wondering what would happen if you did?' Alan hadn't planned on saying that last bit, but as he said the previous sentence he felt that wonder becoming present within him.

'I'll do my best.' Dave was curious as to why Alan had said that, so he asked him, 'What had you in mind?'

'I'm just aware that sometimes an urge to drink can arise quite strongly, sometimes triggered by something that happens, or a feeling or a thought, as you know, but sometimes the urge seems to almost come from nowhere. It can feel quite an irresistible urge. It's a difficult one to deal with. Often if it becomes present then it helps to talk about it, mention it to who you are with, try to talk it out rather than act upon it. The urge to drink can cut in quite fast, almost instinctive, faster than the intellect can rationalise a different response, other than heading off for a drink. Hadn't meant to say that much, but it kind of came to mind.'

Alan knew he had stepped right out of Dave's frame of reference, yet it somehow felt right to have said what he had said. He wasn't sure why. But he trusted this kind of instinct. He was in therapeutic relationship with Dave and he needed to be open to these kinds of thoughts and impressions. He knew things about alcohol that Dave didn't and he felt a responsibility to voice anything that came strongly to mind as it could well have relevance.

'I had some of that the other week, didn't I? Yeah, I'll be mindful of that. I do have those numbers. I am aware things can happen fast but I am feeling different somehow. I'll be OK.' Dave glanced at the clock and was aware that the session was nearly over. Time had passed by very quickly. 'My time's nearly up. So, I'll carry on as I am, keep a track of what I drink and I really want to look at whether I feel in control or not when I choose to have a drink. That seems important. So, can we go for the same time in two weeks and then I can tell you how I've got on. I've got a busy week on at work next week. I also feel as though I have moved on, you know. I do feel much calmer.' Dave was aware of this calmness, which had been present since that previous session. 'It may seem strange but experiencing and naming that fear of failure did something to me. I still don't want to fail, but it somehow doesn't feel such a big deal at the moment.'

'As if you are not living out of that part of yourself, the fear of failing part,' Alan responded, thinking of configurations of self as he said it and sensing that Dave had moved away from his 'fear of failure' configuration into something much calmer and perhaps controlled. But time would tell. It was early days and whilst he hoped Dave would get things together without having further drinking binges, he also knew they could happen. He was also still mindful of the idea of a two-week gap to the next appointment, that whilst it felt OK in some ways, he was also a little uneasy. He decided to hold this for a moment.

'Yeah, I don't want to fail, but I seem more accepting of myself somehow. I'm not sure why I'm saying that, but it does seem to capture something of what I am experiencing. And at the same time I am not prepared to accept using alcohol in the way I have in the past. I think I'm getting more real with myself.'

'I think so too. It's a good feeling, yeah?' Alan replied, wanting to just hold Dave in this natural experience. Then he slipped in a comment that he knew was coming from his own agenda, but he felt this was perhaps a fleeting opportunity to reinforce something important, 'And you don't need alcohol to experience it!'

Since Dave had mentioned the time, Alan had been sitting with the awareness that Dave had wanted to talk about the previous week's experience. 'Dave, you wanted to talk about last week's experience as well but we haven't had time. Is that OK? And I also want to check out again about two weeks to the next session. You really feel comfortable with that gap?'

'Yeah. I kind of do. It is going to be a busy week at work and I do need to be there. We have a couple of training days and I have meetings I have to be at next Wednesday. It's going to mean that I have to be there the other two days. It's how it is. And I also think it would be good for me to have this extra time between appointments. I do feel a lot calmer. But I'll call if I feel different, or if anything happens.'

Alan is having to trust Dave here in a situation where there can be no certainties. Had Dave mentioned it earlier in the session then maybe time could have been used on this, but this was not the case. Dave is making choices and feels he has to prioritise work. Life does not necessarily revolve around counselling appointments. Alan has ensured Dave is aware that he can call if he needs to and he has the helpline numbers.

Alan decided to accept this. If Dave couldn't get away, he couldn't get away, and he did want to encourage Dave to make his own choices. 'OK, you have the number if anything happens, or you want to talk anything through that comes up. And you have the helpline numbers. And you are OK not talking very much today about your experience in the last session?'

'Yeah. I kind of wanted to focus more on the drinking pattern and Christmas. I guess I still haven't really made sense of last time, and yet I know I feel different. Maybe I don't need to try and explain it. Maybe I should just accept it and build on what I am feeling now.' He stood up, and Alan followed his cue. They smiled at each other. Dave then did something that he had never done before in his life. He stepped forward and gave Alan a hug. 'Thanks. Couldn't have done that a few weeks ago,' said Dave as he turned towards the door. 'See you in a couple of weeks.'

Alan was smiling still. Dave really seemed to have moved on, seemed more freed up, more open to his own experiencing. Yeah, he had been on the roller coaster the previous week, but something had shifted from that experience. Could Dave sustain it? Well, it was up to Dave, but at least he felt Dave would get in touch if he needed to. He was strongly aware of his sense that Dave was being more realistic and was more fired up to get his alcohol use sorted.

Summary

Dave arrives late. He is feeling positive and has reduced his alcohol consumption. He is feeling in control and wants to discuss this, along with Christmas, and what happened in the previous session. He only has time to address the first two issues. Alan avoids offering a list of suggestions and Dave begins to come up with his own ideas, and also realises he needs to discuss the planning of Christmas with Linda. Dave decides he wants to maintain his current level of drinking. He is also allowed to affirm to himself that he has experienced a shift and that he feels a lot calmer. He does not think there are any difficulties coming up and because of work his next appointment is made for two weeks' time.

Points for discussion

- What particular difficulties are associated with Christmas for Dave that you can you identify?
- In what ways might the risk of lapse or relapse be minimised in relation to these difficulties?
- Should Alan have been more challenging over the risk of relapse?
- What would the counsellor need to be experiencing within himself or herself to justify stepping out of a client's frame of reference?
- What do you think about the value of 'generalised empathy' as distinct from 'responsive empathy'?

Wider focus

Always be mindful of the Christmas and New Year period as difficult times for people seeking to resolve a problematic drinking pattern. Clients do not always want a goal of abstinence. It is important to work with the client to achieve their goals whilst being open about any concerns that you may have. Where a longer period between contact arises, it is important to ensure that there are other avenues of support or contact available.

Wednesday morning, 20 December

Alan had got the letter through that morning. Dave had spent Sunday night at the accident and emergency unit at the local hospital. The staff there had been told he was getting counselling for his alcohol problem and they had sent a discharge summary through. It hadn't said a lot, but clearly Dave had been drinking heavily, had overdosed, been found by his wife and was admitted overnight for observation. Alan's initial reaction, other than shock, was to wonder whether he had missed anything. Had he overlooked something that could have avoided it happening?

Alan wondered whether Dave would make the appointment. And if he didn't, should he phone? He decided that he would. He felt sure that Dave would appreciate his making contact, as he was sure to be having a rough time.

The receptionist buzzed him to say Dave had arrived. Ten minutes early, Alan noted. He got up to go and meet him. He didn't believe in letting clients wait if he was free. Dave had arrived early and probably for a good reason. He no doubt had a lot he needed to say, or to be with, in the session.

'Hi Dave.' Alan wanted Dave to know that he had heard from the hospital. He didn't believe in keeping quiet about what he had heard, he wanted to be real, to be transparent. 'You've had a hell of a few days at least. I got a note from the hospital.'

Dave felt relieved, and he felt from Alan's tone of voice that he was feeling for him. That felt good. He really wasn't sure what to expect. He had done some stupid things in his life, but last weekend. What a nightmare. 'Yeah, and I don't want to repeat it. I need your help to make sense of it all. I can't believe what happened. It's like remembering some horror movie, but the difference is I was in it.'

Alan held the door open as Dave went in. He wanted to communicate his unconditional positive regard for Dave. 'Cup of tea?'

'Please.' Alan organised it and came in with two mugs.

'So,' was all Alan said. He was aware that Dave might want to talk about what had been happening, or how he felt now, or something else. He felt Dave should choose, so he left it at that.

'Where do I start? I was doing really well. I had kept to the two cans regime when I did drink of an evening, and I was having dry days as well, and I felt good, really good. What possessed me I'll never know. Everything was fine right through to last Friday, and Friday night. But something happened Saturday morning. I don't know what was going on, but I woke up Saturday morning knowing I was going to have a drink, and not just a couple of cans. I *knew* it. And I didn't fight it. It just seemed so reasonable.'

'So reasonable, yeah?' Alan responded, aware Dave had a lengthy story to tell and feeling he wanted to respond briefly to allow Dave to stay with his flow.

'Yeah, so, so reasonable. Didn't say anything to Linda. Well, I thought about it but somehow I found myself convincing myself it would be all right and she didn't need to know. Yet I knew I was going to drink heavily, I knew it. Why? I keep asking myself why?' Dave dropped his head into his hands and sat in silence.

'Why.' Alan said it not as a question, but flatly, a word that captured the struggle that was wracking Dave's tortured heart and mind. He wanted to empathise but not say it in such a way that Dave needed to answer.

'I mean, everything was going well, but Saturday morning I knew I was going to drink. I knew it, and I did nothing about it. You've probably heard what happened next.'

'Only a brief outline, Dave, not all the details. Do you want to talk it through?'

'I need to make sense of it, Alan, I really do. Linda went off with the children at about 9 am, planning to be back around 6 pm. I had helped her get the kids ready but I wasn't really up for it. Felt irritable. She told me that maybe I ought to go back to bed when she'd gone. I did. Slept until midday. Got up, still feeling kind of strange, and still knowing I was going to have a drink.'

'Mhmmm.' Let him carry on as he wants to, Alan thought. Just let him know you are there and listening.

'I went down the pub to watch the match. I just did it. No resistance, just did it. Can't believe it. Met up with some people I hadn't seen for a while, and spent the rest of the afternoon in the pub. Linda phoned on the mobile about 5 pm, and I said something stupid. I must have been drunk by then, and she heard the sounds of the pub in the background. I felt angry and told her I was staying in the pub and would be back when I felt like it. She told me later that she had said she wasn't coming back until Sunday then, but I didn't register that, you know. Carried on drinking. Then went back to a mate's house and drank a bit more. I gather I fell asleep, woke up Sunday morning and staggered back home. I must have got back home to find an empty house. It seems that I drank all the cans I could find, at least empty cans were found around the living room. Can't remember what I felt, but I guess I was feeling lonely. Don't know what happened, next thing I was coming round in hospital. Seemed I'd swallowed some tablets and passed out. My wife had come back at lunch time and had found me, called the ambulance, and that was that.'

Dave sat silently for a moment of two. 'Why, Alan, why? Why did I drink? And why the pills? If she hadn't come home then, I may not have made it. I must have only taken them a short while before she came home. But why, I've never felt suicidal in my life. I wouldn't want to do that, and my kids, they were there when she found me. What am I like? What have I done to them?

He dropped his head back in his hands and the tears streamed from his eyes. 'What have I done to them?' he repeated, shaking his head.

Alan reached out and put his hand on Dave's shoulder. He didn't feel a need to say anything.

'I haven't had a drink since Sunday morning. The thought of it just turns my stomach. I don't want to drink, Alan, I don't want the risk, not any more. I can't risk all that again. But why did I have that urge to drink? I knew I was going to drink, I knew it. I did nothing about it.'

Alan had heard this from other people, almost as though something takes them over, or some part of themselves rises up and grabs the controls. Some people are quite blinded to other choices; others have a dialogue running inside themselves but still seem unable to stop themselves from that first drink, and then things can get so out of control. From the outside it can appear that the person is making excuses, but for the drinker they can feel quite powerless, as though they are living out of another aspect of their structure of self, often a particular drinking configuration associated with some very difficult feeling and memories that have become dissociated.

'I hear how desperately you want to make sense of the why, of what set you up for drinking on Saturday.'

'Yes, I do, but I can't think of anything. I felt OK going to bed. I slept OK. A little restless, but that's not unusual.'

'Any dreams?' Alan asked, knowing he was wondering whether it had been a drinking dream that had set Alan off.

Drinking dreams are a vivid dream experience that leaves the person convinced they have had a drink, feeling all the symptoms of having had a drink and experiencing an urge to carry on drinking. They can be extremely powerful experiences. People report experiencing a hangover, the taste of alcohol and the sense of disorientation that can come from a drinking session after such dreams.

'Can't remember any. Maybe I was dreaming something, but I can't remember.' Dave struggled to remember, as he had been struggling the last two days, but he didn't know.

'Anything you did Friday evening that might have put it in your mind?' Alan asked, wanting to remain sensitive to Dave's expressed wish to know why, and wanting to help him explore various angles on this.

'We watched a film after the children were in bed. Nothing to do with drinking, though. Quite a sad film in many ways. One of those Vietnam War films. Can't remember what it was called. Pretty violent at times.'

'Sad and violent.' Alan replied.

'Yeah. Very sad, Very violent.' Dave spoke slowly and then went quiet. He looked as though he was remembering something.

'Something stand out for you when you think back to it?' Alan asked.

Dave was deep in thought. Alan could see he was thinking. The room seemed to go very quiet, very quiet indeed. Alan felt he should not say anything to break the quiet. Dave was staring ahead of him. Alan knew instinctively that he had connected with something, maybe something from the film. He waited, whilst striving to maintain full attention on Dave.

Dave began to speak. 'There was this one scene. A little Vietnamese boy. The village had been bombed and the helicopters had come in to finish it off. Fire and screaming. One little boy standing with tears running down his face, just running down his face. He was all alone.' Dave went silent again. Alan thought he seemed to be struggling to grasp hold of some feeling towards what he was describing. 'He was the only one left alive. No one was there for him, no one.' He suddenly looked up at Alan. 'What happened to the little boy?'

Alan felt such tender compassion for Dave and for the little boy he had described. He had not seen the film, but he felt that it was being shown in front of him. The atmosphere in the room was so intense. He felt it would sound ridiculous to reflect what Dave had said. He knew Dave was aware that he had heard him. He looked back into Dave's eyes and slightly dropped the ends of his mouth, took a deep breath and shook his head slightly from side to side and slowly blinked.

Dave looked down again. He felt Alan's presence. He was somehow both close and distant. Dave felt so deeply within himself that everything outside of his skin seemed to be fading away. 'What happened to the little boy?' He sat silently again. 'He had done nothing to deserve it.' Again, a silence. 'He was all alone. No one to dry his tears, no one to see his tears. All alone. It must have happened to hundreds of children.'

Tears were rolling down Dave's face. Alan was silent, not just in words but deep within himself. He did not know what to say. No one to dry the little boy's tears, yet he could do something for Dave's tears, and it somehow seemed incredibly important that he did respond to Dave's tears in some way. He leant over and took a tissue out of the box, and reached over to Dave, offering it to him. Dave took it. More tears flowed and minutes passed. Words formed in Alan's head, he voiced them. 'All alone, but you saw his tears, Dave, and you felt them . . . you felt them in your heart and you feel them in your eyes. You know what it is to have tears and to be so, so alone.'

Dave let out a deep breath and began to sob heavily, continuing to take short sharp breaths. He closed his eyes and lifted his head, trying to control himself but he couldn't. The tears kept coming, his breathing continued in short sharp bursts. His head was in his hands now. 'Oh God. Oh God. It hurts.' He shook his head in his hands, pressing his fingers against his closed eyes, as if to try and stem the flow of tears. The flow continued. He looked up again, taking his hands away from his face. The tears were streaming down his cheeks and dripping on to his shirt collar, creating a watery patch both sides of his neck. Dave swallowed and blinked a few times. The tears were hot in his eyes, they burned and they would not stop. He felt helpless against the flood. Alan was handing him another tissue. Dave took it and buried his face in it. Muffled sobs could be heard and the same, short, gasping breaths.

Alan sat with his total attention on Dave, and with Dave. Words were not needed here. Dave needed a companion and he knew that he had one. He did not reach out to touch Dave to try and comfort him. He felt Dave needed to release these feelings without distraction. He did not want to do something to draw him away from what he was feeling and his reactions. He sensed Dave knew he was there for him. Dave was in catharsis and needed to be allowed to stay with it. To do anything that would pull him out before he was ready, before his own inner process required it, would be unhelpful. So he sat quietly, watching Dave and holding him within his own heart. He wanted to hold his feelings of love and compassion for Dave within the therapeutic relationship. They did not need talking about. Deep pain was being released, deep, deep pain.

Dave was in another place in himself, wracked with hurt, the tears continuing to flow, each one seemed to feel like a droplet of pain. Each droplet released a little more of the hurt that he had been carrying for so many years. He swallowed again and this time felt a shift. The tears were easing and he felt his awareness shift. He was more aware of the room, and of Alan sitting opposite him. He looked so concerned, so caring. He really cares, Dave thought, he really cares. He felt the tears welling up again and they burst out again as he buried his head in his hands once more. He took a deep breath again and looked up, blinking at Alan. 'Thank you.'

'It's OK,' Alan replied, giving a reassuring smile. He guessed Dave was thanking him for being there.

'It was the film, wasn't it? Somehow at the time I hadn't connected with all these feelings. It had seemed like a film and I was watching it and though it was upsetting, it didn't trigger this reaction at the time. But I guess it stayed with me, somewhere, somehow. But talking about it now, I wasn't watching it, I was in it, or rather, it was in me.'

'In you?' Alan replied, allowing Dave space to clarify and explore this a little further if he wished.

'That little boy. I knew what he felt, at least, I knew what I felt. I mean, I had nothing like he had to go through. But I knew. I really knew. I understood. I could have been that little boy and for a few moments there I was ... or he was me.' Dave was regaining his composure a little. He took another deep breath and blew it out, looking Alan in the eye. 'Anyone who says counselling is easy needs their head examined.'

Alan smiled. There wasn't much to say to that. 'Yeah, something like that. You've been through it again. Where has it left you now?'

'Strangely calm although a bit wobbly too.' Dave felt different, lighter somehow, but he also felt a little strange, like he hadn't got his balance. Not a physical balance, a kind of emotional balance. He took more deep breaths. They helped. He began to feel more in touch with his body, and more centred in himself. 'That helps. I think I'm coming back now. I couldn't stop the tears, or the hurt inside me. It just rushed up and out. One minute I felt this lump in my throat and heavy weight in my stomach and the next minute I was gone. Have I been carrying that around with me all these years?'

'Does it feel like you've been carrying that hurt for so long?' Alan replied, wanting to allow Dave the opportunity to draw his own conclusion.

'Yes, it does, and I haven't realised it. How can you carry so much hurt, so many bottled up tears for so many years.' He took another deep breath and blew the air out of his lungs shaking his head from side to side. 'I'm glad you're here, Alan, I kind of felt your presence even though you didn't say or do anything.'

'I was glad to witness what was happening for you Dave. It felt a kind of privilege, and quite humbling to be here when you released so much. Thank you for letting me be touched by that little boy, the one in the film, and the one in you.'

'It meant a lot to me when you handed me that tissue. I don't know why, and I can't explain it, but it kind of acknowledged me, made me feel, well, visible, made me feel I was somehow real, that I mattered.'

'I'm glad I did that for you, Dave. At the time I felt I had no words but I wanted to respond. It seemed the natural thing to do.'

'Natural to you. Thanks for doing that and being here. So, what now? At least we've solved the riddle of why I needed a drink on Saturday. But how do I stop it happening again? And why, why did I take the pills?' Dave was looking intently at Alan, clearly wanting an answer.

> Alan knew there was no clear answer. There never was. Dave would have to make a lot of changes, internally and externally, in order to minimise the risk of it happening again. As for the overdose, he felt he needed to help Dave explore this as clearly as possible. Dave had been very frightened by it and wanted to make some sense of it. Perhaps, here in the relative safety of the counselling session, Dave could explore his feelings. Alan wanted to highlight Dave's questions and leave him free to take his own direction, trusting that Dave knew what he most wanted to focus on.

'You obviously want answers, Dave. It seems daft me saying it in a way, and you have been through one hell of a shock, realising you were capable of taking an overdose. It must leave you with so many thoughts and feelings,' he said finally.

'It was the loneliness that got to me. I just have so much sensitivity around it. And it really seems to set off the drinking.'

'Seems to me that you are right, Dave, and that lonely part of you is very much present at times. At some level, or in some area of your psyche, loneliness is very much alive, and it hurts desperately when you connect with it.'

'So do I stop connecting with it? But that won't work, I mean, it will still be there, won't it? I've got to get rid of it.'

'You've got to get rid of that deep sense of loneliness?' Alan offered a straight empathic reflection, saying it slowly to allow Dave to connect more deeply with what was being said, and in the form of a question.

'Yet it also seems part of me. I mean, it's part of who I am. How do I get rid of part of who I am? I'd like to be able to cut it out, but that seems crazy. I mean, I'd be trying to cut out a hole. All I'd end up with would be a larger hole in my feelings.' Dave was looking and feeling perplexed. He hadn't really thought this through, but as the words came out of his mouth he began to realise the craziness of it all.

'So you can't cut the loneliness out. What can you do with it?' Alan replied.

Alan wanted Dave to formulate his own ideas as he felt sure that within him lay the answer to his problem. Dave needed to connect with his own healing process, his own answers. Alan also knew that in Dave experiencing the unconditionally warm acceptance of his lonely self that he, Alan, was communicating, this also had a healing effect. He hoped that Dave would also begin to feel his own compassion for his hurt sense of 'lonely me' which he believed to have self-healing properties. Do you ever really 'work through' something like this, or do you gain the psychological and emotional resilience to carry it once it had diminished slightly through cathartic release and genuine conscious acknowledgement and acceptance of its presence?

'Well, I need to be with people. I need to feel connected to people. I need to feel, oh, I don't know, somehow, yeah, connected to others, and to feel good about it. Yeah, not just any relationship, I need relationships which make me feel good.' Dave sensed a new energy in himself. The words of the last sentence came out with greater intensity. 'Yeah, I need to be with people that I can feel good with, feel confident with, that I can trust.' Dave looked up at Alan. 'Like you.'

'Like me?' Alan replied, wondering what Dave would say next.

'Yeah, like you. I mean, I feel I can trust you and you don't judge me. That's probably the most important thing, you don't judge me.' As Dave said this, Alan could feel a smile inside himself for he knew the power of non-judgementalism as a therapeutic attitudinal quality. And he knew from Dave's own background how much he had felt judged, and therefore a non-judgemental relationship was immediately incredibly powerful and challenging for Dave, challenging his notions and beliefs about himself.

'It's important for you not to be judged, isn't it, Dave?' Alan replied, keeping his focus on what Dave was making present in the relationship between them.

'Too right. I feel freed up somehow, as if I can move a little more freely. I haven't got to keep protecting myself, or at least, I have the opportunity to be a little more honest with myself.'

'Honest with yourself?' Alan was keeping it simple, wanting to just let Dave maintain his focus and his train of thought. He trusted Dave's process. He hadn't a clue where it was taking him, but that was OK. Let Dave find his own way, and find his own truth as to what was important for him in a relationship.

'Yeah, honest with myself. I can accept now that I have a drink problem, and I can be open about it with you. It was strange coming here today because part of me knew you would listen and try to understand what had happened, and accept me and not judge me. But there was another bit of me that really thought you would have a go at me. I kind of knew you wouldn't, but this feeling was around.'

'So while you knew I wouldn't judge you, something inside you was expecting me to have a go at you,' Alan responded, holding both experiences and allowing Dave to be free to choose what to focus on.

'It's that bit of me that could never get anything right. I never knew what I did wrong as a child, but I was always being sent to my room. Looking back now, most of it was for nothing. My mother just wanted me out of sight. But I believed I was doing something wrong all the time. And I still find it hard to take criticism, even when I know it is unfounded. Part of me expects to be judged.'

'Part of you expects to be judged,' Alan replied.

'Dave could feel a new thought coming to mind that hadn't really struck him before. 'Yeah, and if no one else judges me I judge myself.'

'Mhmmm. You judge yourself if no one else judges you. Feels tough trying to avoid being judged all the time.' Alan was struck by a sense of Dave being very much trapped, judgements coming from him from within and without, with nowhere to escape to. 'Feels kind of trapped?'

Dave put his right hand against his forehead and dropped it across his mouth, then rested his chin on it. He blew out a deep breath. 'Trapped, yeah, trapped in my room as a child, and trapped in myself today. This is weird, I was only just saying how I feel freed up to be honest with myself here, and now I'm into feeling trapped.'

Opposite feelings often seem to come together. Entering into one extreme feeling often brings sharply to attention the presence of its opposite. Alan had seen this many times with his clients. And often it left the person craving one thing yet generating the opposite. It was frequently rooted in those early experiences which set up a craving for one experience yet the opposite was becoming introjected as normal. The same drama then gets lived out through life: still a craving for one thing yet the structure of self is carrying a conditioned urge to maintain the opposite. Alan was struck by a question that was playing on his mind. Was Dave feeling trapped in other areas of his life: his work, his marriage, his drinking? Or was his drinking a way of trying to break free from himself? He let the question sit as he heard Dave speaking again.

'But I'm not trapped here. I feel I can talk about whatever I want. But out there, I have to keep watching myself. I can't just be me, whatever that means. Reminds me of something I heard George Harrison, the ex-Beatle say, in an interview they were showing recently on TV. All you need is to answer these questions in life: "Who am I? What am I here for? Where am I going?"'

Alan had also seen that interview and had been deeply affected by it, but was wary of getting into a discussion about it. He had his own thoughts but knew he must push them aside and allow Dave to continue with his own reflection.

'Who are you, Dave? What are you here for? And where are you going?' Alan could feel himself nodding his head slightly as he said this slowly and deliberately, and waited for Dave to respond.

'I'm a mess,' Dave replied, and then sat silently for about ten seconds, and then continued, 'and I'm not a mess as well. I'm determined to get myself together. I've got to. I've got to.' Dave could feel a surge of vitality within himself as he had said 'and I'm not a mess as well'. Somehow instinctively he knew that he was more than a drinking problem, more than his loneliness, more than something small and invisible caught in a trap. He felt kind of warm inside, and somehow bigger.

Alan could feel his perspective shifting, Dave was blurring around the edges, and he felt something deep was going on within Dave. He felt it important to stay really connected and open to impressions, and to whatever Dave wanted to communicate to him.

'I am . . . , well, I don't know but I am bigger than all of this. I feel a real surge of strength.' Dave was feeling and, he thought, probably looking a little bewildered, but something had just happened within him. Somehow he felt distant from the events of the weekend, the film, the drinking, the overdose, the loneliness. He felt strong. He felt good. 'This is crazy but I feel good, and I am aware of what has happened as well, and I want to be sure I can move on from it all.'

'Feels crazy to feel strong in spite of all that has happened?' Alan voiced his response as a question. He really wanted to check out he was hearing what Dave was communicating from within his frame of reference.

'Yeah, and I know it isn't crazy as well. I'm going to beat this, Alan. I really am.'

Alan could hear the determination behind Dave's words. There was a calmness and a power to his words as well. 'I hear the calm but powerful determination in your voice, Dave, you really are going to beat this. '

'But I've got to sort this loneliness out. The alcohol use is a reaction. It is secondary although I know it is a problem. And it took me somewhere on Sunday morning I never want to go near again. That just wasn't me. I had never, ever thought of ending my life.' Dave sincerely believed this and was still shocked by what had happened.

Alan wanted to check out whether Dave really had never thought of ending his life. He believed Dave, and he knew how easy it was to forget things, or discount thoughts at particular times of ones life. He responded, 'Never, ever thought of ending your life?'

Silence. 'Not seriously, I mean, no, not seriously.'

Dave looked disturbed as Alan responded. 'Not seriously? Sounds like you have thought about it, but somehow it didn't seem serious?'

'As a teenager at home I did sometimes wish I was dead, well, no, not wish I was dead, rather think I might be better off dead. Never planned anything, though.

But I did wonder what it would be like to be dead. Couldn't imagine it, somehow. It never happened. That's a stupid thing to say!' Dave smiled. Alan smiled too.

A few moments passed in silence before Alan asked, 'So, no plans to take your life but sometimes you wondered whether you would be better off dead?'

'Yeah,' Dave breathed out a heavy sigh, 'but not all the time, I mean, I didn't carry the idea around with me all the time. Just when I was feeling miserable and sorry for myself sometimes. But it passed. It isn't something I've thought about for years and years. Then Sunday happened.' Dave lapsed back into silence, he was clearly thinking about something and Alan guessed it was Sunday morning and the overdose, or what had come after. He needed to check his assumption.

'Thinking about the overdose?'

'Yeah, yet I don't remember it. I have no memory of what was going on from when we went back to Jim's house for those drinks after we left the pub. Haven't a clue what happened. The next thing I remember was coming round in A&E, with tubes in me and feeling absolutely awful.'

'No memories, like you blanked out the whole experience?'

Alan thought this sounded rather like an alcohol blackout. This is where someone remains conscious and active but drinks themselves into a state of mind in which they seem to store the memories of their experiences during blackout in their brains in some way such that they can't access them when they come out of blackout. It could be very frightening but is also quite common among persistent heavy drinkers.

'Yeah. Nothing. That's scary. I mean, I could have done anything, couldn't I?' Dave looked and felt worried.

'Scares you to think of what might have happened?' Alan replied, holding the focus on the scariness and the idea that anything might have happened.

'I'm sure it was because of how much I had drunk, and then coming home to find no one there, at least, that's how I'm making sense of it now. But I don't actually remember what I felt when I got home. Thank God Linda got back when she did. She's been brilliant. It must have been such a shock to her as well. I gather she phoned me on the mobile late Saturday afternoon to say she was running late, spoke to me in the pub, and I apparently must have already been quite drunk. She told me she wasn't bothering coming back as I was obviously out drinking again, and that she'd be back Sunday lunch time. I think she's going to find it hard to trust me now. I haven't had a drink since Sunday and feel determined not to. I don't trust myself with drinking. I think I need to be off it completely for a while. I need to get my head straight. I've proved the last couple of days that I don't need it.'

'You sound pretty clear on that, Dave. You want to be off the booze completely.'

'Yeah. I was doing well last week, and I know I can get back to that, without the cans in the evening. I just need to keep focused, and I know Linda wants to help. We've done a lot of talking the last couple of days, and we've decided to get a baby-sitter in on Friday nights so we can go out to something together, a meal, cinema, theatre, something. And we are going to try and do more at the weekends as a family. I have to make some changes and these seem realistic.'

Dave had been so relieved that Linda had responded positively. He had felt so awful on the Sunday, so scared when he had heard what had happened, and he really thought he had pushed Linda too far. She had been pretty straight talking, but she had also said she wanted to help him, to try and understand, but that she also had to think of the children. She couldn't have them never knowing what they might find when they got home whenever they went out in the future. He appreciated all of that. He hated himself for what he had done. 'I need to get myself together for the children and for Linda.'

Alan heard alarm bells in his head, and whilst he appreciated Dave's motivation, he knew that so often lasting and sustainable change generally had to be motivated from a desire, no, a need, for the drinker to change *for themselves*. 'You want to kick the booze for the children and for Linda, and I'm sitting here wondering about doing it for you.'

'I suppose it's for me, but my family come first. They are the ones that deserve better.' Dave really didn't think he deserved to do anything for himself. He still felt ashamed, humiliated even, by what had happened over the weekend. It left him feeling very small and insignificant.

'I see, so your family come first, they deserve something better,' Alan reflected.

'Yeah. I'll do it for them. I've got to. I want to be part of this family, Alan. I want my self-respect.' Dave looked desperate. He felt it. Alan saw it as well.

'You really are desperate for this, aren't you Dave. You want to be part of the family and get your self-respect back too.' Alan sensed that Dave had shifted from doing it simply for Linda and the children to doing it for his own self-respect. Dave was claiming his need to overcome his drinking problem for himself. Should he highlight this, or might Dave simply switch back to focusing on Linda and the children if he drew attention to this shift? He decided to let it go, and keep his focus on Dave's perception.

'I've got to. I can't go on like this. It isn't doing me any good, and it isn't doing anyone else much good either.'

'Can't go on in the way that it has been ....'

'No, I've got to go for abstinence, at least for a while. I need to get my head together. I need to start to get a life, get a focus away from drinking.' Dave came in sounding strong, cutting across Alan before he had finished his sentence.

'Sounds really strong, go for abstinence, get your head together, get a life, get your focus away from alcohol.' Alan was touched by Dave's shift to a greater determination. He had connected with his own drive to get himself together.

'The question is how, particularly with Christmas and New Year coming up. Still, if I'm going to do it, I've got to find a way of coming through this time of year. You must know lots of others faced with this situation. How do they cope? What do they do?'

Alan smiled, aware he was feeling pushed into giving advice. However, he really wanted to encourage Dave to formulate his own ideas. And he wanted to acknowledge Dave's request for help. 'OK, so you want some ideas. Of course, what other people have done might not be right for you, but maybe we could just brainstorm a few ideas.'

'Sure.'

'So, what kind of situations are you going to have to handle? When do you think you are going to find it most difficult to maintain abstinence?'

'Parties, I guess. There's the office party and we're bound to be invited round to friends and neighbours, and then we'll have visitors too. Everyone drinks.'

'So, what about we take each situation one at a time? Parties came to mind first, in particular the office party.'

'Yes, well, that always leads to really heavy drinking. I can't see how I can go to it and not risk drinking. I mean, everyone expects you to drink.'

'A real expectation to drink heavily. You can't see yourself going to it without drinking.'

'Yes, I can't go to it, can I? I mean, there'll be a lot of pressure to drink. I'm going to have to come up with a reason not to attend. I need to think about that because it starts with a meal early afternoon and then goes on through the afternoon and into the evening. It's in work time as well so to not attend would probably mean taking a day off. Or do I risk it? No, I can't see myself not having a drink and whilst part of me thinks I could handle one or two, I'm really not sure anymore. I don't want to take the risk. I don't want it getting out of control.'

'So there's a lot of pressure and whilst part of you thinks you could risk it, you also feel strongly that you can't take the risk, that it would get out of control.' Alan felt that Dave was being very open, allowing his internal dialogue to be voiced, and making his own decision as to what was right for him. He was in effect listening to his own internal locus of evaluation, processing his options for himself in order to reach a conclusion that he could feel comfortable with.

'Yeah, I can't see myself not drinking. The best thing I can do is take the day off. That shouldn't be a problem. It's the Friday and I can say that we're going away at the weekend and getting away early.' Dave felt quite relieved at having said that. He hadn't seen this option before. He just thought that attending the party was inevitable with potentially disastrous consequences.

'So, you can't see yourself not drinking if you go, so take the day off and say you're going away at the weekend, is that what you are deciding?' Alan thought it best to respond with a questioning empathic response, which left Dave open to reflect a little more and maybe affirm to himself what he felt he wanted to do. A straight reflection might be experienced by Dave as encouragement and not allow Dave the freedom to explore his thoughts a little more.

'Yeah, missing one office party is not going to be the end of the world. I've got more important things in my life. I don't want to put myself at risk. I'm not going.' Dave felt clear, in fact he felt angry. He wanted to get his life together.

'OK, so missing one office party won't be the end of the world. You've got more important things in your life and you don't want to put those things, or yourself, at risk.' Alan then added, having noted Dave's tone of voice, 'and you sound pretty angry too.'

'Yes, but I'm also scared of slipping up. I was doing really well last week and then it all fell apart. It's horrible. It's like I want to trust myself, but I can't trust myself.'

'You want to trust yourself but you can't trust yourself.'

'No, but I've got to try. I know there are going to be times over the next few weeks when I am really going to feel like a drink, either as a reaction to something happening, or because it is going to be freely available. But I can't drink. I have got to get a grip on myself.'

'So your major risks are with drinking on feelings or drinking because of availability.'

'Yes, and I guess I can do something about the latter, at least to some degree, by controlling where I go and what we have in the house. But the feelings come over me so powerfully sometimes. Part of me wants to get rid of the feelings, but another part of me knows that this won't happen, that I've got to be strong enough to not act on them in the way I have in the past.'

Alan noted feeling good about Dave's last remark. It was very realistic. Yes, it often seems that rather than get rid of sensitivities, you learn to carry them and to make different choices in response to their becoming present. 'So you can to some degree control availability, but you think that the feelings will need to trigger different reactions?'

'Yes, when I feel lonely I have to be able to ... .' Dave lapsed momentarily into silence. 'I was going to say that I have to do something else, but that won't work, will it? I need to accept these feelings as part of me. I don't like them, but they are me, aren't they?'

'You feel you have to accept these difficult feelings of loneliness, they are part of you?'

'I've been fighting them, not too successfully, trying to push them away. But that doesn't work, does it? What a bloody legacy from childhood.'

Alan nodded, allowing him to just be with what he had just said, and waited to see what line he would take next. Dave was certainly gaining a lot of insight in the latter part of this session.

'I have got to move on. What happened in the past was not my fault. It wasn't me that was wrong, that was bad, that was somehow deserving to be punished. My mother was out of order. I don't have to keep replaying it. I don't have to allow it to keep messing me up now. I have got to move on. I have got to do things differently. I have to think about things differently. I have to react differently.' Dave looked Alan in the eyes and said slowly and thoughtfully, 'I have to grow up, don't I?'

'That's how it feels, that you have to grow up?' Alan replied, voicing his response as a question to allow Dave to explore and clarify further what he was meaning. He felt deeply impressed by the work Dave was doing, he really was making some powerful affirmations, and they felt very genuine.

'Yeah, it's my life and I have responsibilities. But I have a lot to learn. I mean, I really struggle sometimes with the children. I can feel quite awkward. I find it hard to play with them sometimes.' Dave went silent again. Alan allowed the silence to remain. Dave continued, 'I didn't have much of a childhood really, didn't have many friends to play with.' He shook his head and took a deep breath. 'This sounds awful, but I kind of feel I sort of lost out on my childhood.' Dave bit his lip, 'So I need to learn to play with my kids. I really want to play a fuller part in their lives, Alan, I really do. And Christmas is a real opportunity for this. Yeah, I'm going to keep away from the booze and get a few natural highs from playing with them. And I'm not going to keep much booze in the house. We haven't much at the moment anyway, but I need to talk to Linda about this. I don't want her to feel she can't have a drink, but I need to talk it through. And I'm going for a quiet New Year as well. That will be different. I want to start the New Year as I mean to go on.'

'Sounds as though you are re-prioritising and wanting to make some important changes.' Alan did not attempt to paraphrase all that Dave had said. It would have left Dave listening to him rather than staying with his own thoughts and feelings.

'Yeah.' Dave sat silently.

Alan glanced at the clock. Dammit, he thought, we are running out of time and Dave hasn't really explored the overdose. Still, he thought, he could have spent time on this and Alan did trust Dave to know what he wanted from the session. He felt he needed to acknowledge Dave's silence but also mention that there was only a few minutes of the session left in case Dave hadn't noticed this to be so.

'Seems to have left you with a lot to think about, Dave, and I am aware that there are only a couple more minutes till the end of the session. You seem to have covered a lot today. I am aware of the one area we haven't talked about which you said you wanted to – what happened Sunday with the overdose. But maybe that's for another time. I think you are in a very different place in yourself at the moment.'

'Yeah, I have to get down to organising Christmas and the New Year. As for the overdose, I know it happened, and I can begin to understand it now. What with the film and the empty house, and the alcohol. It still doesn't seem real somehow and yet I know that it was. But I must move on.'

'OK, now the next appointment will be in the New Year, first week of January. Same time on the Wednesday?'

'Yeah, that's great. It's going to be quite a test.'

Alan was aware Dave was looking troubled and, he felt, understandably so. He would be more concerned if Dave didn't. 'You look troubled, Dave, and I think that's perfectly understandable.'

'I'm wondering who I should tell. I think family and close friends will understand. I want to avoid pressure.'

It is a common question and an important one, particularly at time of family reunion. The people who need to know are those who will be supportive. Those who are going to make it difficult – often those who have a drinking problem themselves that they are not acknowledging – can be told, but in reality they are simply best avoided where possible.

'So there are some people that you would like to tell, that you feel it would help?' Alan noted time was up, but he sensed this was important, and he didn't have another client.

'What do you think?'

'People often find it helpful to tell people they feel they can trust. It can take some of the pressure off.'

'Yeah, I think I need to be open about my decision to be dry for a while, and why. It feels a relief thinking about it, although I wonder how they will react, but then I'm not going to tell everyone, only people who I may spend time with over Christmas, and who I feel comfortable telling. I am also wondering what to do if things go wrong as well. Can I phone the agency?'

'Sure, someone will be here on working days, and there is the local drug and alcohol helpline, the number is on the notice board outside, they are 24 hours throughout. Don't forget you can call a doctor, or if things do get desperate for whatever reason and you do feel you are at risk, there is 999, but hopefully that won't be necessary. And there is always Alcoholics Anonymous, Dave. I know we haven't talked about this option, but they can offer more than anyone in terms of 24-hour availability, meetings and support. It helps so many people, and whilst I know that it isn't for everyone, it is an option. You might want to find out more if you haven't already. That's for you to decide. There are some leaflets in reception in the rack. And there is always the Samaritans. Put the numbers near a phone, then they can be easily found and you'll be more likely to make the call. Let's hope you don't need to. You sound positive, and I think what you have been planning is realistic.'

'Thanks. I hope I don't need any of them. I'm not planning to call them, but it is good to know I can call the Agency and that there are some other points of contact for support. So I'll see you in January and tell you about my sober Christmas!'

'Go for it. I'll look forward to hearing about it, and if there are problems, well, we'll sit down and make sense of them, yeah?'

'Yeah, thanks. See you next year.' Dave got up and moved over to Alan giving him a hug. 'I'm going to do it,' he said. 'Thanks for everything.'

'I'm sure you are,' Alan replied. He was feeling confident. He did feel Dave had shifted profoundly during the session and gained valuable insight for himself. Time would tell, of course, but he was pleased to have spent that extra time so Dave could reflect on whom to tell, and whom to contact if needed.

Summary

Dave has had a lapse into heavy drinking leading to an overdose and emergency admission to the accident and emergency department. In the session it becomes clear that a film triggered Dave into his feelings about loneliness as a little boy. A major cathartic release follows. Alan supports Dave in making sense of what happened. Dave feels a shift occur inside himself, feels a calm and powerful determination to get over his drinking problem. He has recognised for himself that he needs to aim for abstinence, at least for now. He then moves on to plan for the Christmas period.

Points for discussion

- Had Alan missed anything that he could have said or done to have further minimised the risk of Dave lapsing into heavy drinking?
- Emotional traumas leave emotional scars. Do they ever completely heal, or are they always a wounded area that we have to carry with us and build up resilience to?
- How would you feel knowing a client is coming into a session having just recovered from a suicide attempt?
- Should Alan have directed Dave towards a stronger focus in the session on the actual overdose, or was there added value in allowing Dave to direct the session?
- What kind of support do you feel you require in order to work with these kind of issues?
- What other forms of support are made available to people when agencies are closed, or a private counsellor is unavailable, over holiday periods or weekends?

Wider focus

All health and social care professionals have to be clear in their attitude towards lapse or relapse and to overdoses or suicide attempts. They are an all-too-common experience for heavy drinkers. Judgemental attitudes are unhelpful but they are times that can push professionals and leave them emotionally drained, frustrated and stressed.

Friday afternoon, 22 December

'I want to spend time today reflecting on the whole process of working with Dave, and then look at my own feelings towards his attempted suicide, which I need to tell you about and generally talk through, particularly as it wasn't really talked through between Dave and I, and I think some work needs to be done on it for myself. I want to try and get a clearer picture of Dave and of how his self-structure seems to have evolved. I don't have the whole picture, but it seems to me that it would be useful to review and to take stock of the process so far, where Dave is at, and where I am as well. So maybe we can use the time to do this?' Alan was looking forward to this supervision session. He generally enjoyed supervision because it made him think, helped him to get a clearer understanding not only of clients but also of himself in therapeutic relations, and he valued someone else's responses and reaction. So often he felt he missed things, and the relationship with Jan had developed to the point where he really felt he could trust her to voice anything that impressed itself on her.

'OK, so a review session, some theoretical reflections and you say Dave has attempted suicide? So I'm wondering where you want to start?'

Jan could have focused on the suicide attempt, but she knew Alan well enough to trust his own needs, and was sure that he would make time to focus on this. It was always an anxiety-provoking issue, and as a supervisor her priority was to ensure the client was safe. She felt sure they would focus on this during the session but she decided she would highlight it if time seemed to be passing and it had not been addressed. She was aware how review sessions and theoretical considerations could take time. It was always fascinating to reflect on 'theory-in-action', but it could also take attention away from areas that were uncomfortable.

'A lot has been happening since I last saw you. Just before the last supervision session, Dave had attended with Linda. The next session he came feeling very positive. He suggested not coming any more. He felt he was OK and I was really uncomfortable about it. He was asking me directly what I thought and, well, I had to be honest with him. I acknowledged what he had achieved, that he felt in control, but I voiced my concern as to whether he was free of the sensitivities that had been triggering his alcohol use. I really was not at all convinced he was OK, and I remember saying something like "Are you really 100 per cent sure you will be able to sustain control?" It wasn't a fair question; no one can really be 100 per cent sure, and if they are, then they are likely to be over-confident. But he agreed he wasn't 100 per cent sure yet felt he was ready to give it a go, that he was getting a lot of support at home. I then asked him what it was that stopped him being 100 per cent sure. I know I was pushing him, but I just was not convinced and felt it was important to explore it. I think I stepped out of being genuinely person-centred, although I did feel my motivation was coming out of my positive regard for Dave, and wanting him to really think it through and explore what he felt about what he was suggesting.'

'OK, Alan, so what I am hearing is that Dave wanted to stop attending, he thought he was OK but not 100 per cent confident, and you felt that you were pushing him to stop and think about it, or explore his feelings, but it left you concerned you were stepping outside of a person-centred approach.' Jan felt she wanted to leave Alan to reflect on this. It certainly sounded as though he had been directive, yet at the same time he was seeking to be congruent to his own experiencing in response to what Dave was suggesting.

'Yes, and it did have value because Dave then went silent and started talking about his fears – in fact not just talking about them, he was experiencing them. There were some quite long silences in that session. He said that he had had enough about being himself, and he connected with some real motivation to get away from who he had been, from being scared, and settling down, feeling part of the family. There was a lot of anger with himself, as though part of him was angry with another part. The part that wanted to settle down was angry with the part that was the old insecurities – I remember he used the word insecurities. He talked of his fear of facing life without drinking. He really moved into all of this fast. One minute he was all for being better and not wanting to come to therapy, and the next he really had connected with it. He talked about being scared of not having the alcohol to let himself plunge into oblivion – that was how he worded it. It was heavy going. So much fear and despair.'

'I am aware of feeling very alert listening to what happened, and wanting not only to hear more of what was happening for Dave, but also what was happening for you.' Jan was experiencing a very sharp focus and sensed that somehow what Alan was telling her now was extremely important. She did not know why.

Jan is using her congruent experiencing. She knows she is being pushed into feelings and sensations that are connected with what Alan is talking about even though she has no clarity in thought as to what it means. But she is aware that she is sensing there is something in Alan that needs addressing, but it has not yet come to the surface.

'Yes, I think I was on the edge of my seat a little. Dave really was in a desperate place. Then he suddenly said that he knew what he was up against.' Alan suddenly went quiet. Jan picked up a shift in the atmosphere.

'What are you experiencing, Alan, something has changed?' she asked, seeing a look of what appeared to be horror on Alan's face.

'I missed it, Jan. He was telling me that it was fear that he was up against, and one of his fears – I think the first one he mentioned – was fear of failure. That must have been what he connected with when he overdosed. I'm probably not making much sense here, Jan. You haven't heard the story.'

Alan then proceeded to tell Jan what had happened, about the film that seemed to have contributed to setting Dave up for drinking, how he had got home and found no one home. 'You see, maybe it was fear that tipped him towards the overdose, but maybe not fear of loneliness, maybe fear of failure. I can't really say why, but somehow my sense is that this is what it was. He can't remember what happened exactly, and what he was feeling. He said that he guessed he was feeling lonely but he wasn't sure.'

'So your sense is that maybe he overdosed on fear of failure rather than loneliness? I am aware of a wonder which is whether your sense of having missed something is a sense of some kind of failure on your part?' Jan was feeling a little disconnected. Somehow this didn't feel quite right but she couldn't grasp why exactly.

Alan now felt a little confused. 'I don't know. Am I making connections here that are my stuff?'

'Connections that are your stuff?' Jan replied as a question, encouraging Alan to explore and elaborate further.

'Let me think this through. Are you saying that maybe my reaction to Dave having overdosed included a sense of failure on my part, and I am now projecting this on to Dave's motivation to overdose? I need to think about this.' Alan thought to himself and tried to remember how he had felt initially when he heard Dave had overdosed. 'I know I really felt for him. No, that was when I saw him. I first heard about it when the discharge note came through that morning.' Alan thought some more, trying to remember his reaction. 'I think you are right, you know. My reaction was one of "what did I miss?". I took responsibility for what had happened. I blamed myself. Where the hell did that come from? I mean, I would normally want to review the process, and that's why I'm here, yet somehow my reaction wasn't general. I was sharper, more specific, yes, a real sense of having missed something, of somehow being responsible.'

'Sense of being responsible for Dave's overdose?'

'Yes, well I know I'm not. He made that choice, or at least part of him did under the influence of alcohol, but my reaction, that initial reaction as I read the discharge note, was a real sense that I had missed something, or at least the thought that I might have missed something. With some clients it is hard not to feel responsible for them even though I know I cannot be. I do the best I can, and the uncertainty is that you can never be sure if it will be good enough for a particular client. Experiences like this bring all this into sharper relief. But I wasn't responsible, and somehow I think it will prove to be an important part of Dave's recovery. At least, I hope so. I don't want to get unrealistic about it but it did seem to give him even more motivation to want to change, and he seemed more accepting of his lonely sense of self, realising he couldn't cut it out but needed to find new ways of responding to it.'

Jan wanted to check out how Alan currently felt Dave to be. She was aware of her responsibility as a supervisor not just for her supervisee, Alan, but also for ensuring the safety of his clients as much as was possible. She knew that the period after a failed suicide attempt was a risky time and that a further attempt could follow.

'So what state of mind do you think he is in now? The problem with overdose is that for some people they learn from it failing and when they try again they make sure they are successful.'

'I don't think that is where Dave is coming from. He was not carrying an intent to overdose. I think it was the culmination of the amount of alcohol in his system, his feelings of loneliness and/or of failure, and his forgetting that his wife had said they would not be back until later on the Sunday. It really has shocked Dave though. He kept asking why. He didn't seem to be conveying feelings or thoughts of trying again; he wanted to make sense of it. I think he is safe but clearly that particular convergence of experiences put him at risk.'

'Are they likely to happen again?'

'Well, his wife is supportive and they are talking. Dave is not drinking again. I guess you can never be sure but I think Dave realises that he needs to be more careful. But he does seem so strongly motivated to change as well. But like him I am carrying a strong sense of "why?" again. Even though we unravelled the drinking trigger I am back to wondering then whether he overdosed on fear of failure or whether that is my projection, or was it loneliness, or was it something else?'

'Fear of failure, fear of loneliness, or maybe something else?' Jan wanted to keep with Alan and trusted him to be able to sift through his subjective reactions to make sense of what had happened.

'I guess like Dave I don't know. What I did experience was a sense of his wanting to know, wanting to make sense of it. Maybe I have carried that with me, that in some sense I am still carrying a kind of will to make sense of it. We managed to make sense of his waking up with the need to drink because of the film he had watched. So maybe I am feeling something of having failed to make sense of why he overdosed.'

'Is it important for you to always make sense of things, Alan, or is it something about the fact that it was a suicide attempt?'

Alan thought about that. 'I think it's the suicide bit. I find it hard to accept suicide without reason. It seems hard to believe that people attempt it without having a clear reason in mind. It's such a massive decision, but then I also know that people can get into a frame of mind from alcohol use and anything is possible, though my instinct is still that there has to be a reason, a definable trigger. It isn't just the chemicals; there's something else psychological that just gets out of proportion in some way and seems to overwhelm the person in the moment. I can't help feeling that I, we, missed something. That sense of having had enough of being himself that he mentioned a couple of weeks before. Part of him had had enough of the drinking. Could it have been that which triggered the overdose? He got home, drank more and just felt "what's the point", that whilst he had had enough of the drinking he was powerless to change it and went off and got the pills. It is so hard to speculate. Dave wants to know. I want to know. The problem for Dave is that he has no memory of the actual overdose. It seems he was in blackout which makes it really hard to work with.'

'And I am aware of an urge to want to join you and I want to stand back and reflect on this process as it is tempting to be drawn in as well. Sometimes it feels like an energy, or something gets passed down the line knocking us all off focus, and it seems that this need to know could easily seduce me as well. Interesting word to use, "seduce", wonder why I used that?'

'Sometimes alcohol is described as being very seductive, drawing the drinker back again and again for more, proving to be irresistible,' Alan replied, aware that he hadn't really thought about what he was saying. 'It is seductive, warm, moist, and it can be quite gentle, but it can also be hard, burning and belligerent too. Sounds like it has masculine and feminine qualities, not necessarily in that order. I hadn't quite thought of that before. Let's keep with this. I am now wondering which qualities seduce Dave?'

'OK, this is intriguing, and I am also aware that we might be getting caught up in this need to know again which may take us away from something else. But let's go with the flow.'

'The thought that comes to my mind is that in one sense Dave uses alcohol to be one of the group, being with his mates in the pub and I am assuming that is the masculine effect of alcohol, but he also seeks to anaesthetise feelings and discomfort, in extreme he seeks the darkness of oblivion, yet when he talked of that dark pit that time, it actually took him into calmness. Now some would say that is all very feminine, a calm darkness, almost maybe womb-like.' Alan could feel himself wondering where this discussion had got him. 'So, let's keep it simple. Alcohol helps Dave to connect with men, and it helps him to disconnect with feelings.'

'Some might say they are the same. Oops. Sorry about that,' Jan apologised, though finding it hard to restrain a smile.

'Yeah, some might,' Alan replied with a smile as well.

'My sense is that Dave is drinking to experience something important, whether that is a positive urge to experience something in particular, or a negative urge to avoid an experience. But his, let us say, being is making a choice and has done for a while. Is it giving him a sense of self?'

'Well, he certainly seemed desperate trying to cope with the idea of life without it,' Alan replied. Then he also remembered something else. 'He also talked of feeling excitement, that's right, about the idea of having to lose himself to find himself. And he nearly did lose himself with that overdose. Good grief, his use of language really got lived out, didn't it? But I couldn't have seen it that way at the time. It is only now I can put the pieces together.'

'Excitement at having to lose himself to find himself. Do you think this was his whole self or parts of himself?'

'I had the same thought. He wanted to lose the insecure, frightened, fearful, lonely part or parts. He wanted to settle down but he never really defined what this meant and what he expected it to give him. I guess because it is unknown to him. That's going to be hard for him to achieve. He talked in the last session of spending time with his children over Christmas, playing with them, being part of everything. Sitting here now I realise how hard this might be. He aims to have a dry Christmas, a first. But I have no sense of what his childhood Christmases were like.'

'What is your hunch?'

'Pretty awful, I imagine. I don't know, but the fact that he hasn't talked about them makes me feel they are memories to avoid. I could be wrong, but I remember him talking of wanting his son's birthday to be not like his were, or at least I think that's what he said. I imagine he will have similar feelings towards Christmas. He really is living on the edge, Jan. It could swing either way here. I know he is motivated to change, and he is thinking about his drinking and taking practical steps to control it. In fact, he is currently dry and going for abstinence, but it is going to be more than changing his drinking pattern.'

Alan was thinking of how Dave was an example of how complex drinking problems can be. They are so rarely just about drinking. He was aware that this was one of the things that so irritated him. So many people just see a person with a drink problem, and are not prepared to look behind the behaviour and get to know the person who, for whatever reason, is using alcohol. We have to work with the person as much as, and probably more than, their drinking behaviours if we are to help people achieve sustainable change to their drinking (Bryant-Jefferies, 2001), and that takes time, and involves relational depth and commitment.

'Yes, I agree, and I am aware of being stuck with something you said a while ago; it hasn't gone away. It's something to do with his not knowing how to be in the family. Perhaps. I don't know what you think, but I am sitting here wondering whether family therapy might be helpful, both for Dave to integrate and learn relational skills in the family, and for others in the family to be encouraged to interact with him. Or is that a bit extreme? What do you think? You are the one in therapeutic relationship with him.' Jan hadn't planned to mention family therapy but as she was talking it somehow seemed to make more and more sense.

Alan thought for a moment. 'I think you are right, but maybe not yet. I think he needs to be more stable. Maybe couple work would be helpful so that he and his wife can work on their relationship as he works on his drinking and on himself.

Maybe the whole family would come later. That's my initial reaction anyway. But I think it is a good idea. Let's keep that on hold for a while and review it. If Dave gets through Christmas and New Year and seems to be on top of it, then maybe I'll discuss it with him. I don't think he is likely to think of it. I'll listen out for anything he says about how he is interacting with the family.'

'OK.'

'I've just remembered something else. In the last session he talked of not having to keep replaying his past, that his mother was out of order, and that he not only had to think about things and react differently, but that he had to grow up. Then he talked of his difficulty playing with the children. He really did seem motivated. There was something very touching about the way he talked about wanting to play with his children and how he felt he had lost out on his childhood. I really felt for him in that moment.'

'How did you respond?' Jan asked.

'He went on to talk about how he was going to have a different Christmas and New Year, and I never really did respond to the bit about his childhood. He seemed to have moved on. It can be quite difficult when someone says a lot and moves on during what they are saying. Do you try to convey empathy for all that you have heard, or the place that the client has moved to with their train of thought or feeling?'

'I guess it depends on the experience of being with a particular client in the moment.' Jan felt this hadn't really answered the question, but she was aware that she was still with what Alan had said before that. 'I'm still left wondering in what way you were touched by Dave feeling he had lost out on childhood. We seemed to be moving on to another subject and have just done what happened in the session. It got lost. Maybe we can address it here and keep it visible.'

'I felt sadness, sadness for what he had not had. It made me feel humble and grateful for my own childhood, which was so different, so full, and with so much affection shown to me. And of course I had a brother and a sister, so my experience was in total contrast to Dave's. I don't think it was a sympathetic sadness though. I really do have a growing sense of Dave's own sadness, and his determination to move on. And as I say that, I am aware of wondering whether he might need to create a fresh sense of childhood in the sessions, or at least do some kind of play therapy.'

'Sounds good, and it will be for Dave to decide when that might be helpful, of course.'

'Yes, but I will keep it in mind as an option. He may feel a need for it. He may get into it through playing with his children, of course. This is going to be a big Christmas for him. I really hope he comes through it OK.'

'What would OK represent for you, Alan?'

'Well, a couple of weeks ago I would have said maintaining some control over the drinking. I hope he achieves that, but with the overdose, well, I guess the stakes are raised now. I hope he comes through alive. I feel sure he will. He was genuinely shaken by what happened and I do think it may prove a turning point, but only time will tell.'

Jan felt she should check out what arrangements there were for Dave to get help if he needed it. 'What support is there for Dave over the next couple of weeks?'

'He knows he can phone us when we are open and he has the 24-hour drug and alcohol helpline number. He knows he can also call the Samaritans if he feels he is struggling. Of course, there is his GP, or in dire emergency 999. I also mentioned Alcoholics Anonymous as an option.'

'Good, I guessed you would have tried to make sure he had some options. Is there anything more you want to say because I am aware you started by saying you wanted to review the process as we come to the end of the year?'

'Yes, well, I do think Dave has moved a lot. I mean, he has obviously had a lot of difficult experiences since coming for counselling. He originally didn't think he had a problem, then began to realise that he did. He connected with, and we identified, that part of his nature that developed within himself in response to how he was treated as a child both at home and at school. His sensitivity to loneliness has become clear to him, and to me, and his continuing need for friends and to belong. Yet in amongst all the despair and hurt he also seemed to touch some inner state of calm as well, in one of those earlier sessions. So in a sense he really has moved around his self-structure and touched into a number of areas of his experiencing. He had that cathartic reaction as well and then there was the relapse and the overdose, which really has shocked him, and I don't really think we will fully appreciate the depth of that shock for a while. He does realise he has a drink problem now, but he also knows that it is linked to his own conditioning experiences. He realises that he needs to move on, to find his place in the family and to create new elements within his self-structure linked to being a responsible father, playing with his children. No doubt as he changes and develops he will seek new interests and experiences, and what these will be only time will tell.'

'What do you think was crucial in his process so far, and what do you think you have contributed?' Jan asked the question because she felt it would be helpful to identify any key experiences within the processes, and that it would be positive and reinforcing for Alan to own his contribution.

'The session when he came with his wife, Linda. I don't know why, but the way they each responded to the other's hurt was so touching, and somehow I think that made a huge difference. I know things have been difficult since then with the drinking and the overdose, but I was deeply affected by what was happening between them, and particularly the way Dave was tentatively reaching out to Linda. He was trying to connect with, and act out of, a compassionate side to his nature that, well, even as I say it now I can feel tears in my eyes.' Alan got out a tissue. 'Just witnessing them together in those moments, very powerful, a real sign of hope and of something new passing between them.'

'It really touched you, didn't it, and I am wondering what it was that allowed it to happen in that session? They clearly hadn't shared their feelings and experiences with each other previously, had they?' Jan wondered whether Alan had chosen this because he was still carrying hurt from his own relationship break-up and was still sensitive to relational experiences, noted the thought and let it go, deciding she would voice it if it persisted. In the meantime she wanted Alan to reflect on his role as this would help him touch into that aspect of his nature and presence that had clearly been so facilitating.

'I guess they felt safe enough to allow what became present to come through. I had offered them, well I suppose I had offered Dave, enough unconditional warmth and acceptance for him to first of all be in touch with and express his feelings that emerged at the party when they were picking teams for that balloon game. This somehow set the tone and I think enabled Linda to then disclose her memories from childhood and how Dave's actions going down the pub rekindled them for her. So it was my work with Dave that had created enough trust for Dave to feel able to bring this part of himself into the open, both to me and to Linda, and things developed from there.'

'So the climate of unconditional warmth towards, and acceptance of, Dave?' Jan responded.

'Yeah, and I think that for both Linda and Dave it was also about respecting their silences and allowing them to be in their silence. I remember how Dave lapsed into silence and Linda opened her mouth to say something and I shook my head to stop her. Then Dave said how he was always picked last for games at school. And Linda then had tears, and comforted him. And then later when Dave really connected with his feelings and was so tearful and emotional, allowing him to be in his distress, and then Linda responding reaching out to him. When Linda talked of her father going down the pub, getting drunk, coming home and being violent towards her mother, and sometimes to herself, there was another silence, which I allowed to be present. You know, it was holding those silences that was crucial, holding those silences, and being attentive to what was happening. They are still vivid to me. I was so alert, my attention held, sort of finely tuned. It's like in therapy I kind of tune into my clients, trying to be empathically sensitive and responsive, and then there are those key moments where you fine tune, when something is going on and it is as if everything inside of me is striving to register impressions from the client.'

'So, feeling alert and finely tuned in those moments of silence?'

'And in the words that were spoken around the silences. You know, we can underestimate the power of silence both as an experience and as a communication. Sitting here now reflecting on this really puts me in touch with a silent place in myself, I feel kind of still and somehow in awe of the process that Dave and Linda went through, and Dave is still going through. Wasn't it Emerson who wrote somewhere of "the wise silence"? I can't remember, I think it was.'

'A kind of wisdom within the silence, is that what you are experiencing?' Jan asked, noting that Alan was speaking quite quietly and that somehow a stillness had settled in the room.

'I don't know, but I think silence is maybe more profound than we sometimes give it credit for. Sharing a silence, or is it sharing in a silence? I don't know. But being in silence with another person is a deep, deep communication. I mean a true silence, not a silence because no one can think of what to say. A deeper silence that comes out of, yeah, out of knowing that in the moment there is nothing to say. Those are powerful, and I think highly significant when they happen. Yeah, it feels good to connect with this. With all the difficulties Dave has been having it seems slightly strange to be sitting here wrestling with the meaning of silence, yet maybe it is important, and maybe it parallels something of Dave's deeper struggle.' Alan suddenly smiled. 'You know, I had forgotten, that passage I looked up after that session, that line: "Look for the flower to bloom in the silence that follows the storm: not till then". I had forgotten about that. That was about silence. It really was in the air, and it is again now. I wonder what is going to bloom for Dave, and for Linda, in the coming days, weeks, months, maybe years?'

Jan allowed silence to be present, and she smiled. Yes, we create moments, or at least, moments are created within the therapeutic process, important moments in which something shifts, some connection is made, and yet for this to happen something has to be still. What was it Rogers had written, oh yes, about 'moments of movement': 'those moments when it appears that change actually occurs' (Rogers, 1961, p. 130). Yet it always felt to her that within such moments there was a stillness, however brief, when the connection was made and knowledge, or rather a knowing emerged into awareness. Moments when suddenly everything stopped and then, perhaps almost as suddenly moved on, yet somehow profound change and growth had occurred in that brief interlude of stillness, and it could be infinitesimally short.

'I am thinking of Rogers' "moments of movement" and what part silence plays in them,' she said.

'Yeah,' Alan responded. 'They are the magic moments we seek for our clients, yet which we can never *make* happen. The sound of a "moment of movement" is a bit like the sound of one hand clapping. This seems more like "Zen and the art of counselling"! Has anyone written that one? Maybe we should!'

Jan couldn't help laughing. 'Yeah, maybe. OK, so anything else you want to say about Dave today, or do you want to move on to any of your other clients?'

'I think I'm ready to move on to other clients. Thanks for that, for enabling me to connect with the importance of silence. I am sure that it has deep significance for Dave and it will be interesting to see if this proves to be true.' Alan suddenly remembered something. 'No, there was one other important time with Dave, in that last session, when he had a strong cathartic reaction as he was talking about the film that had triggered his drinking. Somehow I think that was a possible turning point as well. It seemed an expression of some really deep feelings. Of course, the one person he has not yet released feeling for is his mother. And that has to happen if he really is going to move on because he must be carrying some powerful and mixed-up feelings towards her. But I guess the time is not yet right for that. Anyway, I am sure that will arise when the time is right and I will trust Dave's actualising tendency to bring that to the surface when the time is right. Let's move on.'

Summary

Alan reviews the previous session with Dave and he connects with the possibility Dave had overdosed on a sense of failure rather than a sense of loneliness. He questions whether this is so or his own projection and this is explored. He also explores his feelings of responsibility for Dave. Jan checks out Dave's current state of mind, aware that once a suicide attempt has been made a further attempt could follow. The meaning of alcohol use for Dave is considered in masculine/feminine terms. Alan goes on to review the whole counselling process with Dave – a kind of reflection at the end of the year. The therapeutic power of silence is discussed.

Points for discussion

- Much of the supervision session will have been taken up with Dave. What criteria would you have for booking extra supervision sessions to deal with client work?
- What do you think about the notion that 'fear of failure' rather than 'fear of loneliness' may have been the primary factor in the overdose?
- Counsellors do miss things in therapy. What is a 'good enough' counsellor? Is 'good enough' an acceptable standard?
- What are your experiences of 'moments of movement'? What process underlies their becoming present in a session?
- Would you want Jan for your supervisor? Discuss your perception of her strengths and weaknesses.

Wider focus

What kind of supervision and support are professionals other than counsellors offered in order to deal with clients offering such complexity as Dave and to enable them to disentangle their own emotional and psychological content from the client's process?

Wednesday morning, 3 January

It was only after the supervision session that another thought had struck Alan. He had found himself wondering how much Dave was projecting on to Linda, particularly given the strength of his reaction when he thought she might have abandoned him that Sunday morning, leaving him in the house on his own. Was she likely to be the one that would trigger his release of feelings for his mother? He felt that perhaps couple counselling might be helpful sooner rather than later to help this to be worked through, as clearly the feelings would be strong and could be quite devastating. He decided to raise the issue of couple counselling with Dave during the next session, as the more he thought about it, the more it seemed appropriate and necessary.

Alan had not heard from Dave over Christmas or New Year so he was hoping that everything had gone well. Dave was due in a couple of minutes and Alan was sitting in the counselling room being with his thoughts and feelings.

> When he could, he liked to take some quiet time before a session, to get himself centred. What did this mean? He saw it as first of all being in touch with himself and then gradually slowing down his breathing and letting himself relax whilst at the same time seeking to be consciously aware of his senses. He felt it was important to prepare himself before meeting clients so that he could try and be present for them as fully as possible and without other concerns, which could be set aside, being carried into the therapeutic relationship. Of course, this could never be completely achieved. Thoughts or feelings from outside the therapeutic relationship would arise but he hoped to be able to identify them and ease them to one side and keep focus on his client and his own experienced responses.

His mind wandered back to the previous supervision session and the recognition of the importance of silences. Counselling sessions may last 50 or 60 minutes, but there were moments that somehow seemed more important when he really had to be as fully present and congruent as possible. He also wondered what Dave might have experienced over Christmas. He knew it was fruitless to speculate and fill his head with expectations. He wanted to be clear and open to whatever Dave brought to the session. Two weeks. So much could have happened. Unlike some counsellors, he was not too bothered about remembering all the details of the previous session. A mind full of memories would obstruct him in the present session and whilst information could be useful to inform, it could also stop him initially being fully open to being in relationship with Dave as he would be today. Dave was not the same person who left the counselling session two weeks ago. He would have undergone whatever experiences came his way over Christmas and New Year. He, Alan, had no idea what these were and what effect they might have had. He needed to be fluid enough to connect with Dave today, not the Dave he still carried memories of from two weeks ago.

Time had passed and Dave was overdue. Ten minutes had passed and Alan began to feel concern. Just as he got up to check that there had not been a message that he had missed, the receptionist buzzed the intercom to say Dave had arrived. Alan went out to greet him and to bring him back into the counselling room. He looked well, Alan thought, but he wasn't going to express this. He had fallen in that trap before, telling someone how well they looked only to get blasted by a client fed up with people saying that when they felt like shit inside.

'Hi Dave,' Alan began, 'good to see you again. Come on through.'

'Thanks, and Happy New Year,' Dave responded.

'And to you,' Alan replied.

'Sorry I'm a few minutes late. Bit hectic this morning with the children around.'

That's OK. I was getting a bit worried. So, where do you want to begin today?'

'Well, it has been interesting. Before New Year I would have been able to say quite proudly that I had kept in control, which I had. The odd glass of wine and can of beer, but nothing over the top, and no major problems. At the parties I stuck to non-alcoholic drinks. I actually found myself watching people and realised that somehow I didn't feel left out. In fact Linda and I sat "people watching", and I think because we had each other to talk to and be with I didn't feel left out or anything. I actually realised how much rubbish people were talking as they got more and more drunk. I actually felt quite glad to feel sober! That was a first.'

'So, a sober party spent with Linda "people watching", and somehow the two of you being together helped you not to feel lonely and therefore at risk of drinking alcohol?'

'Yeah. I felt good. Even remembered the party next day!' Dave went quiet for a moment, pondering on the experience. 'I am sure it was because of being with Linda, being a bit like we used to be, you know, kind of close. It felt so good. I didn't feel a great need for a drink. It really has shown me that I drink on loneliness and feeling left out of things. I didn't have those feelings at all, and I didn't drink. Of course, had Linda not been there, well, who knows, but she was and it has given me a lot to think about.'

'So, it has really sharpened up your realisation that you drink in loneliness and feeling left out. And you are also left wondering how it might have been had you been there on your own.'

'Well, I think I probably wouldn't have gone on my own. In fact, it was deliberate that we went together. I had been uneasy about it and I talked it through with Linda and she agreed to come along, and that we would work at it together.

I said she could drink but she said no, she would stay sober too. I actually think that helped.' Dave had been really pleased with that evening and he and Linda had become closer as the evening wore on. They had made love when they got home and it had really felt like the old days.

Alan was aware that Dave had gone silent and seemed to be in his own thoughts. 'You look as if you have drifted into some memory, Dave, and it seems to be making you smile.'

'The evening really brought us closer together and we had a wonderful night together when we got back. Makes me realise how important our relationship is to me. But then there was New Year which, well, I drank more than I intended and Linda did get rather worried, but it was only that night and I haven't had anything since. We went out to a dinner dance and we had a bottle of wine with the meal. I then had a few beers and, well, I seemed OK but when we went outside to get the taxi I lost it. Must have been the cold air I suppose, but I really had trouble standing up. We got back OK, and I guess I must have slept it off, but I woke up next morning with an awful hangover, which I don't usually get. Linda wasn't too impressed and it wasn't an easy start to the day. We didn't exactly row, but we didn't say a lot either. I did feel awful, couldn't really motivate myself to do anything. Fortunately, it was a holiday so I didn't have to go to work. We began talking about it late in the morning and decided that maybe we ought to go out in the afternoon, get out the house and try and put the evening behind us. We ended up going to the coast with the children. Walked along the sea front. It wasn't too bad, bit cool but dry and sunny.'

Alan felt he didn't want to interrupt Dave's flow, so in the pause he simply responded with a nod and an 'Mhmmm, afternoon at the coast with the family. How was it?'

'Fine, we talked a little although we couldn't say too much with the children around. Maybe that was a good thing as it kept us focused on them. We ended up in the amusement arcade for a while and that was fun and we all came out smiling and had hot doughnuts.' Dave was aware that he had a lump in his throat and could feel tears in his eyes. Alan had noticed his watery eyes too.

'You look really affected by that, Dave.'

'Yeah, I just felt so part of the family, you know. It just felt good, having fun, having a few laughs, and the doughnuts were brilliant. Made me realise what I wanted.'

'What you wanted?' Alan asked, allowing Dave the opportunity to elaborate if he wished.

'To really feel part of the family. I felt proud as we walked along, the kids running around us. So much energy. They never seem to stop, do they? It just felt good and I want more of it. It made me realise that I have missed out on a lot. Linda often took the children out with her in the past. Whenever we went out together we would often end up sitting in a pub somewhere, or I would and she would take the children around. I've learned a lot the past two weeks. It hasn't been easy, but I was determined. It was only New Year's Eve that I messed up.'

'So, you have realised that you really want to be part of the family, and that you drink on loneliness and feeling left out. You have realised that you have missed out on a lot and are determined to change that.' Alan was struck by a sense of warmth for Dave. He felt good hearing what had happened and pleased that New Year's Eve had not triggered off major problems. He guessed that a lot had to do with Linda's reaction. Had they argued the next morning it could have been very different.

It reminded him how important the reaction of a partner is when someone lapses. They can't always stop the lapse happening, but they can certainly contribute to the lapse becoming a full relapse. But it was never easy for the partner of a heavy or problematic drinker. At times it didn't matter how they reacted, it could always be turned into an excuse by the drinker to go in search of a drink. So many partners carried stress, were anxious and depressed, their lives so affected by not only the drinking but also the unpredictability of their drinking partners' reactions to any comments made. Problem drinkers could be so sensitive to criticism, however valid it might be. The drinking behaviour could so dominate the family that the needs of the person drinking could be lost sight of. In the tension, the person and their thoughts and feelings could get lost, leading to isolation and the urge to drink more.

He also recognised that a partner could deliberately sabotage someone's attempts to stay sober or in control as a way of gaining power. He had seen some pretty strong, sometimes violent, power struggles of this nature. There were often some powerful co-dependency issues to be addressed although how many times had he heard it said to him that the non-drinking partner didn't want to be involved in anything, they were OK, they didn't have the drinking problem.

'You look miles away, Alan.'

'Sorry, I was just thinking about how partners are affected by a heavy or problem drinker and how difficult it can be.'

'Yes, I now realise something of the impact I have had on Linda, particularly given her early life experiences with her father. It really shocked me when she talked about that when she came here with me that time. I just never knew. Well, I had no reason to. I still drank heavily New Year's Eve, though, and she had to help me up the stairs and into bed. I'm not surprised she was off with me the next morning. I'm lucky she didn't react even more.'

'Yeah, that was kind of part of what I was thinking about, how important a partner's reaction is to someone when they have a lapse like you did.'

'It could have been a lot worse and I am grateful that things worked out and what started a really awful day actually ended up really good. Just that makes you think.'

'Makes you think?' Alan asked, again hoping to encourage Dave to explore this a little more.

'Well, we could have ended up not speaking all day and I don't know what I would have felt or done. I'm sure it would have put me at risk of drinking. I'd have felt isolated and lonely and anything could have happened. Or Linda could have been really critical and, well, threatened to go out on her own or something. That really would have been hard to stay sober with. But she stuck with me and it turned out OK. I'm grateful for that, and I don't want to push my luck. I mean, I know she loves me and I love her, but I'm sure she has a limit. I don't want to push her to that limit and risk everything. My marriage is too important to me. I really know that now. The thought of … no, I don't want to think about it. I want to stay positive. I have done well and I want to build on it for this year.'

'You don't want to think about what might happen if it all went wrong. You want to keep a focus on the positive achievements and build on them.'

'I do, but I also know I am carrying that sensitivity to loneliness, and I have to deal with that. I have to somehow become more resilient. I kind of have to avoid those feelings . . . .' Dave stopped and thought for a moment. He heard Alan say 'Avoid those feelings?' 'Well, I can't really avoid them, but I need to respond differently to them. Alcohol isn't the answer. I know that. I've got to take a different path, somehow, and I feel I've made a start. Being with the family more, being closer to Linda again, that feels like a different path. And maybe it needs other features as well, you know? We talked about new interests in one session. I really need to run with that. I'm not sure what, but I do need a fresh start. Otherwise, the old pattern is kind of waiting for me, isn't it?'

'That how it feels? If you don't take a different path then you are at risk of going back to how it has been?' Alan was aware that a passage from a book had come to his mind, and it seemed to really sum up where Dave was at. It was something he always had a few copies of in case it felt right to offer it to someone. It felt right to offer it to Dave.

'Yeah, like avoiding a hole in the road by going down another road.'

Alan smiled. If that isn't a nudge he didn't know what was. 'You ever come across the passage about the hole in the pavement in a book called *The Tibetan Book of Living and Dying* (Rinpoche, 1992)?'

'No.'

'Well, it goes like this and I can give you a copy if you like it.' Alan shuffled through his papers and pulled out a sheet:

1   I walk down the street.
     There is a deep hole in the sidewalk.
     I fall in.
     I am lost … I am hopeless.
     It isn't my fault.
     It takes forever to find a way out.

2   I walk down the same street.
     There is a deep hole in the sidewalk.
     I pretend I don't see it.

I fall in again.
I can't believe I'm in the same place.
But it isn't my fault.
It still takes a long time to get out.

3   I walk down the same street
There is a deep hole in the sidewalk.
I see it is there.
I still fall in ... it's a habit.
My eyes are open
I know where I am
It is *my* fault.
I get out immediately.

4   I walk down the same street.
There is a deep hole in the sidewalk
I walk around it

5   I walk down another street.

Dave sat for a moment, 'Oh yes, I need a copy of that, oh yes. That's it, isn't it.
That hole, but it isn't in a sidewalk, it's inside me. It's about me being different,
me getting out of the habit of being the me that I was, and becoming ... well
becoming something else.' Dave's eyes were very watery again. He had been
deeply touched listening to that passage. That hole was familiar, and he had
to accept responsibility for falling in it, and he had to make choices to keep
away from it as well. 'Where do I find the other street, Alan? Have you got a
map?' Dave laughed as he asked the question, although behind the humour
was a serious question.
Alan sensed this, 'No map, but it is a serious question, isn't it?' he replied.

Alan was aware that they had previously talked about Dave's relationship
with Linda and he hadn't said anything about couple counselling, but the
thought was back with him again. He knew he was introducing something
from his frame of reference, yet he genuinely felt it was worth exploring.
Couple counselling could be helpful, but he also felt that it would need
a counsellor who had worked through his or her own attitudes towards
alcohol use.

'Dave, the thought has been with me as to whether you and Linda would find
some kind of couple counselling helpful, to help you build on what you have
achieved. It may not be necessary, I sense you are both keen to make the relationship work, but I just wonder whether it might be helpful.'
'Funnily enough, we had talked about it, and whilst we haven't made a definite
decision – it would need planning to make time with the children as it would

have to be evenings, regularly in the daytime would be difficult. But we are talking about it. That session when we both came to you made a deep impression on both of us and helped us to be a little more open, though I know I still had that awful weekend and the overdose and didn't feel able to tell Linda how I was feeling. But yeah, we are talking about it. Where can I get names of people who would be credible?'

'You may be able to access it through the NHS if your surgery has a counsellor offering it. Otherwise there is Relate. Also you might want to contact the British Association for Counselling and Psychotherapy who have a directory of registered counsellors. I can give you their address after the session.'

'Thanks. I'll talk to Linda again. Anything that helps me, and us, avoiding that hole in the pavement.'

The two of them lapsed into a silence. Somehow it felt as though the session had ended although it was early.

A thought came back to Alan's mind. The issue around fear of failure that he had discussed in supervision. He had had it in mind right at the start before the session began but the session had taken its own direction, and he felt that this had been right. Should he raise it now? But Dave had been in blackout and did not know or could not recall exactly what had triggered the overdose, what feelings had been present. He was mindful that there was a risk of false-memory syndrome here as well. He didn't want to introduce something that Dave then took on board and adapted his understanding around. He hadn't thought of that in supervision. Damn. Yet, as he was thinking about it he felt he could not just ignore it. It would be hard to justify, he thought to himself, particularly if a problem arose linked to this and he had not drawn attention to it. In extreme it might even be regarded as negligent, and in an increasing litigious society .... No that was certainly not a reason to raise it. It had to be a genuine congruent expression of something present that was felt to be relevant to the relationship with Dave. He felt he had to trust that it had come to mind for a reason and that this was relevant to the relationship he had with Dave as it was in this moment.

'Dave, something came up in my supervision and it is back with me now because I think it might be linked to the overdose. I guess I need to check this out, and I think it would be inappropriate not to mention it. The fear of loneliness that we identified as a possible trigger. I found myself in supervision wondering whether there was also a "fear of failure" around as well.'

Dave sat and thought about it for a moment. 'Somehow, it all seems a bit distant now. Fear of failure. I'm not sure. You mean failure with my marriage?'

'Not sure what I mean specifically, it just came up as a theme and it just came back to me. Maybe talking about couple counselling brought it back into my mind, so perhaps that's the connection. I don't know.' Alan was aware he was doing a lot of talking and Dave a lot of listening. Maybe it wasn't relevant after all and it had been his issue.

'I don't want my marriage to fail, and at the moment, I mean, OK we had our problem New Year, but it feels positive and I am feeling optimistic.' Dave was slightly taken aback by this fear of failure stuff. Had that been what he had felt? He just didn't know.

'Seems like it isn't relevant, Dave, and while I kind of felt I needed to raise it, I'm also feeling sorry I raised it.' Alan now wished he hadn't said anything.

'No, that's OK. I don't know what happened and maybe one day I'll get some insight into it. At the moment I guess I'm open to suggestions.'

'Open to suggestions,' Alan repeated, 'I guess what I don't want to do is to put suggestions into your head that really can't be substantiated within your experience.'

'Yeah, but it does make some sense as I think about it. I mean. I never felt I was good enough, you know, and so it's a feeling that has to be around. It's whether it was active that Sunday morning. Maybe I'll never know. But perhaps I need to keep it in mind and accept that both loneliness and failure could be triggers, and that if they come together then I really have to watch out. I really don't know, Alan. And I also want to remain positive as well. I've got through Christmas and New Year, and the coming year is an opportunity to make a fresh start with a renewed sense of optimism. I do feel different. Something definitely shifted in that session before Christmas. I want to move on. I want to get things together at home, you know? I don't think I'll ever forget what happened, but I'm not sure that I want to dwell on it either. I want to move.'

Alan sensed the strength of feeling present. 'Yeah, you want to move on.' He smiled. OK.

The session came to an end and Alan felt pleased that Dave had come through Christmas with a positive experience and that the New Year difficulty appeared to have been resolved.

Alan knew he had to take this fear of failure issue back to supervision but probably more importantly into personal therapy. He had felt the need to voice it to Dave, but the moment the words were out it just felt as if he and Dave were wading through treacle with it. Maybe it was around for Dave, but perhaps he had voiced it from his own stuff and not out of a genuine sensitive response to something present within Dave. If it had been present for Dave as well in some significant measure than maybe it would have felt different. Perhaps if there was something in this for Dave then maybe it was a case of bad timing, that it needed Dave to be more fully in touch with it, which was not the case at present.

Summary

Dave describes his Christmas and New Year experiences. He has realised how important it is to feel part of the family. Dave realises he needs to find a new direction or new path and avoid the pitfalls linked to his past and his alcohol use. Alan raises couple counselling and Dave informs him that they have thought about this. He feels that things are moving on in a positive manner. Alan introduces the 'fear of failure' issue that was discussed in supervision and it doesn't really feel appropriate once the words had been said.

Points to be discussed

- What would you see as the key advantages in couple counselling and what would you expect to be the major themes that would emerge in this case?
- In an increasingly litigious society, how much does this damage a therapist's ability to be transparent and spontaneously creative within the ethical boundaries of the therapeutic relationship?
- Would you have raised the 'fear of failure issue' and if so, how? And if not, why not?
- What is your reaction to the 'walking down the street' passage? Was it appropriate to introduce this and, if so, what is the theoretical justification?

Wider focus

Introducing ideas that are not from the client can be fraught with difficulty, and in particular where the client genuinely has no memory of something. The risks of false-memory syndrome are widely recognised in relation to child abuse, but it has validity to alcohol blackout and other traumatic experiences where memory has been disturbed or lost.

Wednesday morning, 17 January

Dave arrived on time. He was feeling good, much clearer, much more positive and in control. He knew he still had a long way to go, but he also felt that his life was changing and that he was making choices that were much healthier for himself and his family. It was strange how he had adjusted. It felt that he was creating new aspects of himself, new identities within his personality. He no longer had a social life that was pub-centred in the way that it had been in the past. He was looking for new interests. He had joined a sports club and was enjoying getting a little fitter, although it was a struggle and he had found a few muscles that he didn't know existed. They were doing more as a family and he felt a strange sense of belonging, which now, in hindsight, he realised had not been present for him. With this had also come more openness in his marriage, more ability to not only be aware but also to share his thoughts and feelings with Linda. They were talking about so many things, but most of all about themselves. Yes, he felt good, he felt positive, but he was not complacent. He wasn't too sure what he wanted to talk about today, but that didn't matter. He seemed far more able to accept the uncertainty. It was sure to throw up something of interest and relevance. It always had done in the past.

'So, how do you want to use our time today?' Alan asked as he sat down opposite Dave.

Dave thought about it. 'I don't know. I'm feeling good. I am amazed how different I feel.'

'Feeling good and amazed how different you feel?' Alan intonated his reflection as a question to invite Dave to explore further.

'I was just thinking that it feels as if I am becoming a new person. Well, not completely new, but as though I am discovering, or am I creating, new parts of myself. It's hard to put into words, but I'm different. I'm realising that I can feel good in making new choices. I still have an occasional drink, glass of wine with a meal, occasional pint with a pub meal, but I'm not dwelling on it, thinking about it. It feels like I have moved on. And at the same time I am aware that it was only a month ago when I took those pills and everything was crazy. But that seemed to be a turning point.' Dave had strange, mixed feelings. He hated what had happened and yet somehow it seemed to have been a blessing in disguise. It had kind of pulled him up and forced him to rethink so many things about himself and his life. It had sharpened up his awareness of what he wanted, and what he wanted to leave behind.

'So, a feeling of newness and a realisation that the overdose was some kind of turning point?'

'Seems so. I mean, I guess I still carry those sensitivities that have triggered heavy alcohol use, particularly the loneliness, but I am taking steps to fill my life with experiences that make me feel a part of things. It's as though I am off-setting the sensitivity, building myself anew. It seems to be releasing a whole lot of energy. I could even call it a different kind of energy if that doesn't sound too odd.'

'You feel a different kind of energy?'

'I just feel more enthusiastic, more willing and able to engage in life. I'm taking more of an interest in things. I'm even enjoying my work more and I feel a greater urge to progress.'

Alan felt excited by what Dave was saying. 'It feels tremendously exciting listening to you talk about feeling, what comes across to me, as being more energised.'

'That sums it up; you've hit the nail on the head there. More energised.'

'Mhmmm,' Alan replied nodding his head and waiting to see where Dave wished to take the session.

'Feels good.' Dave paused. 'How many sessions have we had now?' he asked.

'Twelve sessions I believe. Any reason that you ask?'

'Part of me feels that it has been a long process; another part of me feels that time has gone by so quickly. It seems strange to have both feelings at once!'

'So, both long and short.' Alan added what he was experiencing. 'It has felt to me to be long in the sense that so much has happened yet short in the sense that we have actually spent less than 12 hours together in this room.'

'It is strange. These short periods of great intensity and then back out there. It has been an interesting journey to say the least!' Dave allowed himself a smile, to which Alan responded with a smile too. 'And it isn't over yet, is it?'

Alan felt his eyebrows rise. 'Does it ever end?' he asked, then realised that he had slipped into a more philosophical frame of mind and had left Dave's frame of reference.

'I guess it doesn't, but I would like to think I can move on from the whole alcohol bit.'

'You would like to think you can move on.' Alan kept to a straight empathic response to help Dave stay with this thought if he wished to.

'Yes, I do, and I know I can but when I say that, I know as well that I am not being complacent. I am sure within me that the loneliness button, and maybe that fear of failure, still lurk. But I want to focus on building myself up, creating a fresh sense of self.'

'OK, I hear you acknowledging those sensitive areas whilst also wanting to create a fresh sense of self,' Alan replied.

'I do.' Dave sat silently for a moment, and something from an earlier session came back into his head. 'I am just remembering how in an earlier session I was talking about cutting out that loneliness, and recognising that that was kind of impossible. But it is part of me, isn't it; it is something of who I am? I can't deny it, I can't get rid of it, but I can surely choose another way, like in that passage you gave me last time. It is not just a different outer path I have to take, but an inner one as well, isn't it? I not only have to avoid the hole out there, which is drinking. In fact that may not be the most important hole. The really important one is the one in me. That's what I have to avoid. And yet there is also a feeling that avoiding it may serve me for a while, but it still isn't the final answer. I have to fill the hole in, and then I can freely choose which path to travel on.' Dave felt himself feeling, well, the only word he could think of was *integrated*. He felt he was somehow coming together, feeling more complete somehow.

Alan sought to check out that he had heard what Dave was saying correctly. 'So, there is an inner hole and an outer hole. The outer hole is drinking; the inner hole the feelings that drive you to drink. You see a need to avoid the inner hole by walking down another street, but you eventually need to fill that hole so you can make a genuine free choice without fear of falling in the hole again.'

'That's right. I can either avoid my feelings, or . . . the words that come to mind are, make them safe.'

'Make your feelings safe,' Alan replied with a hint of question his voice, inviting Dave to explore more if he wished.

'I'm not sure what I mean. I'm kind of talking out my own thoughts here as they come to me. But it is about being safe.' Dave stopped for a moment, and then added, 'and being secure'.

'Safe and secure,' Alan replied.

'If I can be that then I can move on from it all.'

'So your sense is that feeling safe and secure will enable you to move on.' Alan was aware as he said this that he wasn't too clear exactly what this meant in terms of Dave's drinking. Did he mean that he felt he could drink without it causing problems, or was he still looking to be abstinent?

Dave answered this in his next comment. 'I can move on, get my life together, stop living out patterns from my past. But I will still need to watch the alcohol use. I know now that once it gets into my body to a certain level it can affect my thoughts and feelings. I do seem OK to drink the odd glass of wine or beer, but I need to watch it. I know some people cannot, that one glass seems to lead to another and another and another. I think that is the same for me when I am drinking on certain feelings, but I am lucky that when those feelings are not behind my choice to drink I can take it or leave it.'

Whether someone overcoming an alcohol problem has to remain abstinent or can drink in a controlled manner is a huge discussion point. Some take the view that once you have a drink problem and have the 'disease' of alcoholism, you must remain abstinent. Others think more in terms of problem drinking as a learned behaviour, which can be changed and/or controlled. Added to this is the genetic factor which researchers continue to investigate. Is there an alcoholic gene? Or are genetic factors more likely to leave people with particular chemical and emotional sensitivities that simply heighten the risk of alcohol becoming problematic? Certainly, prolonged alcohol use does generate chemical changes that leave people more susceptible.

Alan's view was that you had to treat each person as an individual, and that people had their own sets of genetic inheritance, learned behaviour and meanings which shaped their choice whether or not to drink alcohol (or 'use' alcohol), that needed to be understood. He knew people who did not seem able to tolerate any alcohol without it leading to more alcohol use, although he felt sometimes this was because they had not truly dealt with underlying issues. He also knew people who had overcome a drinking problem and were now drinking but in a non-problematic style. It did seem the length of time someone had been drinking heavily was a critical factor, but he also knew, particularly for binge drinkers, the feelings, thoughts and memories they were drinking on were the major factor. One thing that Alan felt strongly about was the lack of social and political commitment to promoting the need to treat alcohol with respect.

'So what I hear you saying is that you need to continue treating alcohol with respect and being mindful of what is behind any given urge to drink. Is that how it is, or am I putting my own meaning into your words?'

'No, that's how it is. And I am sure there will be difficult times ahead, and maybe I will have heavy drinking sessions in the future, though I hope not. I feel like I have looked over the edge of an abyss, actually not so much looked over but at times it is like walking over it on a rope, you know, like a tightrope walker. But that doesn't happen so often these days. But I know it could arise again and I need to be ready for it.'

Alan knew he was smiling because the image had reminded him of a passage from a book he had read many years ago. 'Reminds me of something I read years ago in a little book, "They will ask thee how to traverse life. Answer: Like crossing an abyss on a taut string – Beautifully, carefully, and fleetly" ' (Agni Yoga Society, 1953, p.159).

'I guess I need to learn how to walk that way as well!' Dave smiled. 'Though I would rather not be on a taut string all of my life! But maybe I don't have to. Maybe I can find the right choices to keep myself away from the kind of problems I was having towards the end of last year.' Dave stopped and thought for a moment, and Alan let him stay with his thoughts. He believed that empathy wasn't just about responding to what the client was communicating; it could also have a contextual or situational element as well. Dave was silent and thinking, and he, Alan, would show empathy for that by allowing the silence to continue. After a couple of minutes Dave spoke again. 'I am going to have to deal with that loneliness you know. But I'm not sure whether I need to engage with it again like I have done in the past. But I also know it is powerful. I feel caught between whether to focus on rebuilding myself, or whether to focus on resolving what is already part of me.' Dave paused for a moment and then added, 'It seems like a choice between the old and the new.'

Alan appreciated this comment. It really summed up a key question in therapy that had no easy answer. Do you look backwards; do you address the present; do you look ahead to the future? So often counselling seems to be thought of as looking back, yet he knew that this was not what all clients wanted or needed. His own feeling was that you trusted the client's process, their own actualising tendency, which would bring to attention whatever needed attending to. However, crucial to this was the certainty that a genuinely therapeutic relational climate was being offered with congruence, empathy and unconditional positive regard present as fully as the therapist could manage.

Alan recognised that he was not an expert on Dave's inner process. But he felt he could trust it to take Dave to where he needed to be. It seemed that often the therapist's congruence encouraged the client's incongruence to the surface of their experience. Alan certainly felt that congruence was a key factor working with this client group.

As ever, the future was unknown. People change, they move on both inwardly and outwardly, and it is important to trust them to know what is most present and pressing for them.

'Whether to focus on the old feelings of loneliness or the new feeling that you are building into yourself.'

'Yeah, and I don't know. I somehow feel I have to trust myself here, my own inner wisdom, and I also know that whatever I do there will always be risk.' Dave shook his head slightly, acknowledging to himself that it all seemed a bit of a mystery to him.

Alan could hear himself thinking a phrase that he was sure someone had said Rogers, the founding father of person-centred therapy, had used, but he didn't know if this was true and, if so, where it came from. He voiced it anyway. 'Life is a risky business, yes?' He added, ' You feel you want to trust yourself, your own inner wisdom.'

'I can dwell too much on problems. I don't think that's good for me. I want to emphasise the positive, the achievements. It's not that I want to deny difficulties, but I don't want to over-focus on them. I guess there will be times when I will do, and I have to trust that these occasions will be timely for me.' Dave smiled. 'Here am I saying all these things, and how long have I felt in control of my drinking, just a few weeks!'

Alan sensed that somehow Dave was putting himself down and he wanted to respond to this because he felt it important for Dave to be able to acknowledge that he had his own wisdom and that perhaps he needed to listen to that more. It also sounded like Dave was in the process of shifting his locus of evaluation (Rogers, 1951) from an external to an internal focus, from being shaped by the opinions of others to a trusting of his own reasoning, feelings and inner promptings. He wanted to acknowledge this but without getting into technical terms.

'I hear you saying you want to trust your instinct to focus on the positive, to trust your own inner prompting and insights, yet another part of you seems to be trying to undermine this. Both are aspects of you.'

'They are, and I do want to trust my own instincts. That somehow seems really important. I know they haven't always been trustworthy. Remember when I wanted to stop coming, and when I felt I had got control of my drinking. Both times you were right to be uneasy and to voice this, though at the time I had convinced myself I was OK. But it feels different now. I don't feel I am having to convince myself. I feel more open to who I am and I want to trust this "who I am". That probably sounds really weird, but it is where I am in myself.'

'I hear you loud and clear, Dave, you want to trust yourself, your "who I am".'

'And in many ways I do, but in other ways I know that I don't. And maybe that's how it has to be.' Dave stopped. 'Maybe that's how it has to be,' he repeated quietly to himself, 'sometimes I can trust myself, and at other times I am not so sure.'

'Sometimes you feel trusting of yourself, other times not so trusting,' Alan replied, keeping his empathy to a simple, straight reflection to allow Dave to develop his thoughts and feelings.

'I don't trust the bits of me that have been hurt. I don't trust the people who have hurt me.' He stopped and thought. 'I find it hard to trust people, Alan. So many have rejected me in the past. Somehow I don't think that you will reject me though.'

'OK so the way you see it is that you find it hard to trust people, particularly those that hurt you, and you believe that I won't reject you.'

'Yes.' Dave was silent again, thinking about it all. He suddenly spoke slowly, 'I make people reject me too, don't I?'

'You make people reject you?'

'Well, I've been thinking about this a lot over the last couple of weeks. And I think I do. I mean, my drinking provoked Linda into rejecting me in a way, and it seems to me that part of me feels rejection is natural. And I see this as linked back to my past. And part of me accepts being rejected, and another parts hates it, or it's maybe the same part that both accepts it and hates it. I don't know. But I am also experiencing a growing urge to not want to accept it any more.'

'So, let me check out that I am hearing you accurately. Part of you has normalised rejection and that part also hates it. And you are experiencing an increasing urge to reject your acceptance of rejection?'

'Reject rejection, yeah, that puts it quite nicely. And there is anger in there too. Anger towards those who taught me to feel this way, who gave me the feelings and experiences that left me feeling rejected and alone.' Dave's voice was suddenly stronger and louder.

Alan was wondering if this was heading towards a release of feeling for Dave towards his mother. Anyway, not for him to speculate, stay with him, maintain empathy, congruence and unconditional positive regard. He responded, 'anger' deliberately lifting his voice and making it sound strongly affirming. He didn't say anything more. He didn't need to, and besides, single-word empathy whilst sometimes difficult was often powerfully effective. Usually the tone in which the word was spoken was at least as powerful as the word itself, and sometimes more so.

'Fucking angry. I can see the faces of the kids at school. I guess they weren't to blame. They were just being kids. I'd already learned to accept rejection by then. No, it wasn't them to blame. They came along after the damage had been done. No, the real cause of it all was my mother, and my father who I never really knew. My father buggered off when I was three and, well, you know what happened then. Bloody crap childhood. Hours and hours in that fucking bedroom, on my own.' Dave could feel the fire in his belly and the energy filling his whole body. He slammed his fist down on the arm of the chair. 'Years of it. Bloody woman hadn't got a fucking clue.'

Alan kept his response short to allow Dave to continue, '... not a fucking clue'.

'No. And I am sick to death of feeling what I feel as a result of it all. I've had enough of carrying it around with me and it buggering up my life in the present. I never see her these days. We haven't had contact in years and I'm bloody glad. I've got my own life to lead, I've got responsibilities to shoulder and I need to feel confident, and I'm going to be. For fuck's sake, Alan, I've bloody well had enough of it all, and I'm damned if I'm going to let her mess up the rest of my life. I've had enough. I'm moving on and ... ,' Dave stopped, he was clenching his knuckles and his eyes were blazing.

'You've had enough and you're moving on.' Alan was aware he was nodding his head and very aware of the shift in atmosphere in the room. It felt electric.

'How could she fucking well treat me like that, Alan? What the fucking hell had I done to her? And I want to be bloody angry about my father, but that's harder 'cos I can't remember him the same. I can't think of him. I haven't got a clear image or memory. He's just this shadowy bastard that buggered off. Obviously didn't give a damn. Never heard of him again and bloody well don't want to. Fuck them both.' Dave took a few deep breaths and shook his head. He could feel the anger welling up inside him like hot, molten lava. He clenched his fists again and looked at Alan. He breathed out powerfully and shook his head again. 'I've never spoken like this about them before, Alan, but I really needed to. I've been holding on to all of this. I'm bursting with it.' He got up and paced up and down the room. 'Ahhrrgghh! Bloody hell. How do I get rid of all of this, Alan?'

'Feels to me like that is precisely what you are doing now.'

'Yeah, I bloody need to.' Dave walked over to the window. He breathed in deeply and blew out his breath with an explosive force, pausing briefly before taking another deep breath to be followed by the same ritual. He looked up at the ceiling and blew out another deep breath. 'I don't think I've ever felt this way before. I feel so, so . . . full of energy. I feel so alive. And so fucking angry.' He clenched his teeth and slammed his fist on to the windowsill. 'Bloody hell!' He turned to look at Alan and shook his head.

Alan sensed there was more anger to come, that somehow it was still not really being expressed. He looked at Dave. 'Hard to know what to do with all the anger and the energy, huh?' And he added, purposefully putting fuel on the fire, 'the bastards'.

Dave clenched his fists again and looked round the room. He slammed his fist down on the windowsill again. 'This is what I have been missing all my life. I mean, I've got angry when drinking, or about drinking, or to give myself a reason to go drinking, but this is different. This is . . . personal. This is me, me, the little boy sent away to his room finding his voice. But this is also me the man. This is different. This . . . fucking hell, this is me. You know, Alan, nothing is going to be the same again after this. I can feel a great weight taken away from me. I feel strong. I feel good. I . . . .' Dave looked up towards the corner of the room and stood silently for a minute.

Alan was aware Dave had stopped himself in mid-sentence. So he reflected it back, 'I,' and waited.

'I don't know, I've not felt this way before, well I have, but not in a way that I could really be aware of myself. Shit, what I wanted to say was, "I feel a man".'

'I feel a man,' Alan reflected back and waited.

'Yeah. Like I've been trapped in childhood or something, I don't know. I've got so many thoughts and feelings flying around, but I feel like a man. Yeah. The feeling trapped we talked about before. I was trapped as a child, and I was stuck in the fucking trap all my bloody life. Well not any more.'

'You feel you've been trapped all your life, but now no more.' Alan felt it important to keep his responses simple and to the point. He had to keep in Dave's frame of reference and let him go the distance with this release.

Dave blew out a few breaths. 'Trapped, but not any more. No wonder it has felt good the last couple of weeks, getting out to do different things. I am moving on and leaving the past behind, Alan, where it belongs. I don't have to live out all that crap anymore.'

Alan nodded

'I needed that. And I needed someone to witness it, Alan. It wouldn't have been the same on my own. Thanks for being here.' Dave walked back to his seat and sat down slowly and thoughtfully, in marked contrast to how he had got up. He shook his head again and tightened his lips, breathing out as he did so. 'They've got a lot to bloody well answer for. But I'm not going to let them fuck up my life any more. They are history for me, it's all history. I can't turn the clock back, I can't forget what happened, but I'm not going to carry it with me any more.' Dave relaxed a little and blew out another deep breath. Alan noticed his shoulders drop. 'I feel drained, but it's a good drained. My head is buzzing. I feel lighter somehow.'

'Lot of strong feelings, Dave, lots of strong feelings of anger, and now you're left feeling drained, buzzing and lighter.' Alan was feeling pleased this had happened in a session. Dave looked calmer now. Where the session would go now he did not know. He knew it would continue where it needed to and that he would let Dave direct it according to his sensed needs and experiencing.

In fact the rest of the session was spent more quietly. Dave described how he felt having released that anger, and wondered whether he had released all that was needed, or whether there was more to come. He said that he thought there was probably more, but he wasn't sure. He was in a sense breaking new ground in terms of his own experience of himself. The session drew to a close with an agreement to continue fortnightly and review after four more sessions and then discuss what further contact and focus might be helpful. Dave also agreed to begin to attend an alcohol support group one evening a week.

By the time Dave left he was feeling more centred. He was certainly looking forward to life ahead of him and in a way that was a new experience. He knew he still had much to learn about himself and was sure that there were going to be a lot of character traits that he would need to face up to. But he felt positive. It had been a torrid few months, and he hoped that he had put that behind him. As he walked away from the building towards the park on his way over to work he was smiling. He didn't know what was ahead but now he felt ready to face it, to learn from it, determined to be a more open and responsive person. He realised that more than anything else he was feeling secure in himself, it was a good feeling, deeply satisfying, and he was ready to explore further who he was and the person he could become.

Summary

Dave continues to do well, feeling in control of his alcohol use and making and sustaining positive, healthy choices for himself. He reflects on rejection and it leads to recognising that he provokes rejection. This in turn leads to an explosion of pent up anger towards his parents, which Alan allows Dave to release, and indeed encourages him to release. The session continues with Dave reflecting on his feelings and whether there is more anger to express. Both he and Dave reflect separately after the session has ended and Dave has left.

Points for discussion

- What do you think about Alan's view regarding whether people with alcohol problems need to be abstinent, or can successfully maintain a controlled drinking pattern?
- What are the advantages and disadvantages of labels such as 'alcoholic' or 'problem drinker' compared with 'a person with an alcohol problem'?
- How would you have responded to Dave's anger?
- Was it therapeutically helpful for Alan to 'throw a little more fuel on the fire'?
- Do you feel optimistic or pessimistic about Dave and why?
- Critically evaluate Alan as a counsellor. Would you recommend him to a friend?

Wider focus

People need to release anger, and professionals in caring professions need to be able to facilitate this. Not only does the professional helper need to feel comfortable with this, but the work setting needs to be appropriate as well. Many settings have paper thin walls that can inhibit emotional release, making effective therapy difficult.

Final reflection

As Dave left the session, Alan reflected on the journey so far. Dave had been through a lot. He had achieved much. He had managed a dry Christmas and New Year, and that was no mean feat in a culture that associated this time of year so strongly with alcohol. He was gaining a great deal of self-insight, too, and was learning to become much more part of the family. He was looking to develop new interests, and hopefully new friends would develop out of that, building his confidence. Of course, nothing is ever certain when dealing with an alcohol habit. Dave had experienced lapses and knew how fast the urge to drink could cut in, and how irresistible it felt. These might well arise again, and only time would tell whether Dave would be able to make other choices in those crucial moments.

He anticipated many more sessions with Dave, much of the time focusing on ensuring that he was maintaining his change, but also exploring with him the effects of his childhood on the development of his self-structure. He hoped Dave would want to continue to attend, to really help himself to redefine who he was, within the support and safety of the therapeutic relationship. He was glad, too, that Dave had elected to join an alcohol support group. In his experience, being with others who were facing up to their own alcohol problem could be very helpful. Not everyone felt comfortable in groups. Often clients did not give themselves enough time to find their way, finding reasons not to attend at the first sign of discomfort or anxiety. Another factor with groups is that you can't easily fool other drinkers. They've been there. They know the excuses. And they are often very quick to challenge. But groups do help people. Alcoholics Anonymous is a group approach and it has proved to be enormously successful for vast numbers of people. However, not everyone feels this is for them, and they may then benefit from a different group approach.

So Dave was moving on, learning a new way of being in the family, and new responses to situations and experiences that touched into the sensitive areas that had been generated so long ago in childhood. Would Dave maintain abstinence, or would he go back to drinking? And if he did return to drinking, would he go back to the old pattern or would he be able to maintain control and keep to social drinking? This has always been a big question and it can generate heated debate. For Alan, where heavy alcohol use was not ingrained over many years and the psychological/emotional factors that drove the urge to drink were being resolved, then social drinking or controlled drinking was much more likely to be sustainable. But even then there was no certainty.

He wished Dave well. He had made the first step. He was no longer drinking in the destructive manner that had become such a habit. He had made the second step. He was no longer thinking much about drinking. Yet he knew life had a habit of throwing up the unexpected and this would be the true test for Dave. Alan allowed himself to smile. At least Dave was on the road to recovery. He was giving himself a chance. He hoped that it would prove to be a sustainable path for Dave and knew that he was looking forward to continuing to work with Dave and be part of the journey.

References

Agni Yoga Society (1953) *Leaves of Morya's Garden, Book One.* Agni Yoga Society Inc, New York.

Bozarth J (1998) *Person-Centred Therapy: a revolutionary paradigm.* PCCS Books, Ross-on-Wye.

Bryant-Jefferies R (2001) *Counselling the Person Beyond the Alcohol Problem.* Jessica Kingsley Publishers, London.

DiClemente C and Prochaska J (1998) Towards a comprehensive, transtheoretical model of change: stages of change and addictive behaviours. In: W Miller and N Heather (eds) *Treating Addictive Behaviours* (2e). Plenum, New York.

Frances L and Bryant-Jefferies R (1998) *The Sevenfold Circle: self awareness in dance.* Findhorn Press, Forres, Scotland.

Knapp C (1996) *Drinking: a love story.* Quartet Books, London.

MC (1920) *Light on the Path.* Theosophical Publishing House, London.

Mearns D (1992) On the self-concept fighting back. In: W Dryden (ed.) *Hard Earned Lessons from Counselling in Action.* Sage, London.

Mearns D (1994) *Developing Person-Centred Counselling.* Sage, London.

Mearns D (1998) *Working at Relational Depth: person-centred intrapsychic 'family' therapy.* Paper presented at the Joint Annual Conference of the British Association for Counselling and the European Association for Counselling, Southampton, September 1998.

Mearns D (1999) Person-centred therapy with configurations of self. *Counselling.* **10**: 125–30.

Merry T (1999) *Learning and Being.* PCCS Books, Ross-on-Wye.

Miller WR and Rollnick S (1991) *Motivational Interviewing: preparing people to change addictive behaviour.* Guilford Press, New York.

Prochaska JO and DiClemente CC (1982) Transtheoretical therapy: towards a more integrative model of change. *Psychotherapy: Theory, Research and Practice.* **19**: 276–88.

Rinpoche S (1992) *The Tibetan Book of Living and Dying.* Rider, London.

Rogers CR (1942) *Counselling and Psychotherapy.* Houghton-Mifflin, Boston, MA.

Rogers CR (1951) *Client Centered Therapy.* Constable, London.

Rogers CR (1957) The necessary and sufficient conditions of therapeutic personality change. *Journal of Consulting Psychology.* **21**: 95–103.

Rogers CR (1961) *On Becoming a Person.* Constable, London.

Rogers CR (1963) The actualizing tendency in relation to 'motives' and to consciousness. In: M Jones (ed.) *Nebraska Symposium on Motivation.* University of Nebraska Press, Lincoln, NE.

Rollnick S, Mason P and Butler C (1999) *Health Behaviour Change: a guide for practitioners.* Churchill Livingstone, Edinburgh.

Thorne B (1985) *The Quality of Tenderness.* The Norwich Centre, Norwich.

Velleman R (2001) *Counselling for Alcohol Problems.* Sage, London.

Velleman R and Orford J (1993) The adulthood adjustment of offspring of parents with drinking problems. *British Journal of Psychiatry.* **162**: 503–16.

Further reading

Alcohol

- Association of Nurses in Substance Abuse (ANSA) (1997) *Substance Use: guidance and good practice for specialist nurses working with alcohol and drug users*. ANSA, London.

- Cantopher T (1996) *Dying for a Drink: a no-nonsense guide for heavy drinkers*. The Book Guild Ltd, Lewes.

- Cooper DB (ed.) (2000) *Alcohol Use*. Radcliffe Medical Press, Oxford.

- Floyd MR and Seale JP (eds) (2002) *Substance Abuse: a patient-centered approach*. Radcliffe Medical Press, Oxford.

- Plant M (1985) *Women and Alcohol: contemporary and historical perspectives*. Free Association Books Ltd, London.

- Plant M and Cameron D (eds) (2000) *The Alcohol Report*. Free Association Books Ltd, London.

- Plant M, Single E and Stockwell T (eds) (1997) *Alcohol: minimising the harm. What works?* Free Association Books Ltd, London.

- Velleman R (2001) *Counselling for Alcohol Problems*. Sage, London.

Person-centred

- Fairhurst I (ed.) (1999) *Women Writing in the Person Centred Approach*. PCCS Books, Ross-on-Wye.

- Kirschenbaum H and Henderson VL (1990) *The Carl Rogers' Reader*. Constable and Company Ltd, London.

- Mearns D and Thorne B (1999) *Person-Centred Counselling in Action*. Sage, London.

- Mearns D and Thorne B (2000) *Person-Centred Therapy Today*. Sage, London.

- Natiello P (2001) *The Person-Centred Approach: a passionate presence*. PCCS Books, Ross-on-Wye.

- O'Leary C (1999) *Counselling Couples and Families: a person-centred approach*. Sage, London.

- Rogers CR (1980) *A Way of Being*. Houghton-Mifflin Company, Boston, MA.

- Wyatt G (ed.) *Rogers' Therapeutic Conditions: evolution, theory and practice*. 4 vols. PCCS Books, Ross-on-Wye.

Useful contacts

Alcohol

Alcoholics Anonymous
General Service Office
PO Box 1
Stonebow House
Stonebow
York YO1 7NJ
Tel: 01904 644026
National helpline: 0845 769 7555
Website: www.alcoholics-anonymous.org.uk

Alcohol Concern
Waterbridge House
32–36 Loman Streeet
London SE1 0EE
Tel: 020 7928 7377
Email: contact@alcoholconcern.org.uk
Website: www.alcoholconcern.org.uk

Drinkline
Tel: 0800 917 8282
Drinkline provides information and advice to anyone concerned about sensible drinking. Callers can be put in touch with local specialist services. Calls are free and do not appear on your bill (except for mobile phones).

National Institute on Alcohol Abuse and Alcoholism
6000 Executive Boulevard
Willco Building
Bethesda
Maryland 20892-7003
USA
Tel: 301 443 3885
Website: www.niaaa.nih.gov

Scottish Council on Alcohol
166 Buchanan Street
Glasgow G1 2NH
Tel: 0141 572 6700

Person-centred

Association for the Development of the Person-Centred Approach (ADPCA)
Email: adpca-web@signs.portents.com
Website: www.adpca.org
An international association, with members in 27 countries, for those interested
in the development of client-centred therapy and the person-centred approach.

British Association for the Person-Centred Approach (BAPCA)
Bm-BAPCA
London
WC1N 3XX
Tel: 01989 770948
Email: info@bapca.org.uk
Website: www.bapca.org.uk
National association promoting the person-centred approach. Publishes the jour-
nal *Person-centred Practice* and a regular newsletter *Person-to-Person*.

**Network of the European Associations for Person-Centred and Experiential
Psychotherapy and Counselling (NEAPCEPC)**
c/o SGGT
Josefstrasse 79
CH-8005 Zurich
Switzerland
Tel: (++41) 1 271 71 70
Fax: (++41) 1 272 72 71
Email: office@pce-europe.org
Website: www.pce-europe.org
Network within Europe of national organisations that promote person-centred
and experiential psychotherapy and counselling.

Person Centred Therapy Scotland
Tel: 0870 7650871
Email: info@pctscotland.co.uk
Website: www.pctscotland.co.uk
An association of person-centred therapists in Scotland which offers training and
networking opportunities to members, with the aim of fostering high standards of
professional practice.

World Association for Person-Centred and Experiential Psychotherapy and Counselling
Email: secretariat@pce-world.org
Website: www.pce-world.org

Index